The Owner's Manual for Health and Fitness Vol 1

Author Credits
Photographer-Charlotte Brown, Models-Rashida Webb and Katie Carpenter

ISBN: 978-0-9863723-3-9

Honor the past......

Learn from the past....

But focus on the future and who you want to be.

George Dorsey

Table of Contents

Acknowledgments

To God...First and foremost, I would like to thank God. Because without God, nothing in my life would have been possible.

To my Mom...Second, I want to thank my mom. She's always supported my efforts even when others didn't. Thank you for showing me at an early age that I can do anything that I put my mind to.

To my Grandparents....I want to thank my grandparents Reverend C. E. Strickland (deceased) and Maxine Strickland (deceased). They both showed me what being a man was really about. More importantly they taught and showed me how to genuinely care about people from all walks of life no matter where they may have come from.

To my Aunt...I want to thank my aunt Rosalind Morrison for her support and for being such an inspiration to me. Thanks for all you do.

To the Skulpt Fam....Last but certainly not least, I want to thank the Skulpt Inc. team, particularly Jose, Juan, Stasia, Gerry and Gonzo. You all helped to give my journey even more meaning. Love you guys!

Preface

So why should you read this book? Well as you can see there are a number of health and fitness books within arm's reach of this book and you can access even more books with just a few clicks on the internet. So what makes my book any different from the others? Of course simply for the fact that I wrote it (That was a joke by the way.), there are a number of reasons that separate my book from other health and fitness books.

Let me present the first reason as a question. Why is the rate of obesity and the waistlines of your average person still growing? The answer to this question becomes even more important when you add that the average consumer is bombarded with messages and information about the latest fitness fads, which are being marketed by the most well-known fitness personalities and celebrities. Now-a-days you have a broad range of people, from psychologist, surgeons and even housewives, all trying to sell you their fitness pitches. So, what are we missing? The reason that we blindly pursue these Pied Pipers of Fitness is because just as the fictional character filled the ears of the children of Hamelin with an attracting harmonious tune, marketers of today's bestselling fitness fads and products, know how to play a similar tune. Now before my phone starts ringing off the hook, I'm not suggesting that all companies, celebrities and fitness personalities are out to intentionally mislead you. What I am saying though, is that you need to do your homework, especially since those who are not in the fitness industry might not quite understand just how this harmonious melody of greater fitness is going to affect their bodies. A lot of the health and fitness information that we see on television or read in magazines are packaged as sound bites, which are meant to get you to buy, not to educate. The focus of this book is to educate. The information in this book is packaged to help you to easily understand basic concepts and principles of health and fitness.

Let me tell you a story. I had a client by the name of Lizzy, (her real name is being hidden to protect her identity). Lizzy had purchased every fitness gadget or fad that has ever been on television. When Lizzy opened her kitchen cabinets or closets at home, they resembled the shelves of Dick's Sporting Goods, the fitness section of Walmart and almost the entire store of Whole Foods. Well not really, but you get the idea. Lizzy stored everything from raspberry ketones to the latest installment of high intensity training workout videos. Unfortunately, even after shelling out hundreds of dollars, Lizzy was still gaining weight and the high blood pressure and diabetes that Lizzy was fighting, were winning the war.

Unfortunately, scenarios like this play out all over the world and people are losing battle after battle. With my book, I aim to clear up this confusion so that a basic understanding of how the body works, how nutrition plays a significant role in maintaining good health and how to develop basic exercise programs is plainly communicated. There is also a section in this book that aims to dispel the many myths about health and fitness that are spread through water-cooler chat, social media and television.

There are many health and fitness books that are written as if once size fits all. Others are written in such a way that the intended message of the book is lost in high level rhetoric and medical jargon. As a military person, I believe in communicating information based on the principles of K.I.S.S. For all you military and ex-military folks you know exactly what this acronym stands for. For those that don't, I'll tell you what it represents. It stands for Keep It Simple Stupid. Now I'm certainly not trying to call anyone stupid. But the premise behind this acronym is that there is no reason to make things or situations complicated, when one can merely use plain English or simple concepts to ensure the reader fully understands the message being conveyed.

Lastly, the prosperity of any economy is dependent on the health and welfare of its labor force. Economic theories tell us that the most prosperous economies have found a way to maximize the use of its workers, machines, factories, and technologies in order to reach the highest output levels for goods and services produced. Adam Smith, in the Wealth of Nations, even argues that "A nation's wealth was to be judged by the total value of all the goods its people produced for all its people to consume".[68] If this is the case, then doesn't it make sense for a nation to ensure that all labor force participants are healthy?

Unfortunately, when it comes to healthcare, large disparities exist between those who have access to healthcare and health information and those who do not. These disparities lead to unequal access to healthy food, medical care, medicine, recreational facilities and health and fitness information.

The National Healthcare Quality Report, a report mandated by Congress, highlights the significant disparities in access to healthcare and the quality of healthcare given, between racial groups.[69] Additionally, several studies, including a study led by Johns Hopkins University, found that residents of minority, rural and low-income neighborhoods had greater access to energy dense foods and foods that promote unhealthy eating, which are mainly served by fast food restaurants and convenience stores. The studies also found that these neighborhoods had limited to no access to supermarkets and other places where residents can find healthy food.

Several studies have even honed in on the effects of poor nutrition on worker productivity. One study showed that Chinese female cotton mill workers who received iron supplementation for several weeks demonstrated a 5% increase in gross and net energy efficiencies, significantly reduced heart rates, and a 17% increase in production efficiency. Other studies have found that iron deficiency affects an individual's aerobic capacity, endurance, energy efficiency and work output. Iron deficiency in children also has a negative impact on their cognitive ability and their ability to produce. Those with higher incomes and higher disposable incomes tend to invest more in human capital. Higher income earners have better diets access to health information, improved sanitation, and better healthcare.[70] Simply put, a healthier worker is less susceptible to disease, is more alert, more energetic and will more than likely be more productive and earn higher wages.

The aim of this book is to arm people from all walks of life with much needed health and fitness information to help fight the war against diabetes, obesity, cardiovascular disease and other preventable health related diseases.

SO WHY THE BOOK TITLE?

I'm a gadget person. I love technology just as much as the next person. I'm always trying to get the latest fitness gadgets, home electronics or the latest smart phone. Unfortunately, one of the first mistakes that I tend to make when I buy a new product, is to throw away the owner's manual, thinking that I'll just figure things out as I start to use the product. Just as usual, I'll read a magazine or see a television show demonstrating all the wonderful features of the product that I just bought; features that would have made my life a whole lot simpler had I just read the owner's manual.

Well, this same thought process holds true when people think about their body. I've come to realize after 22 years in this industry, people think that over time they can just figure out the best way to being healthy. By the time things are somewhat figured out, it is often too late. At least with a product, if you are dissatisfied with its performance, you can either replace it or buy something different altogether. We don't have these options with our body. Also, even if you haven't quite figured out the operational nuances of your new product, you can always refer to the owner's manual to get you on your way. As humans, we don't get owner's manuals when we are born. I mean really. Wouldn't it have been nice, if your mom or dad, just handed you a nice leather bound owner's manual at the age of 10 and told you that the manual contained all the information that you needed to know about how to keep your body fit and healthy? Because we don't have such a manual, we are dependent on our friends, relatives, doctors and health professionals, if you can afford them, to help us to figure things out. Often times, we still don't get it. What type of world do you think we would live in, if everyone had their very own owner's manual for their body? Do you think that the number of people with high blood pressure, cardiovascular disease or diabetes would be anywhere near the numbers that we see today? Probably not.

With this book, I aim to turn back the hands of time. Just think back to the feeling that you had when you purchased your favorite technological gadget. There was joy, excitement, curiosity and an expectation that this product would fill every void that you hoped it would. By reading this book, I hope to bring back those same feelings, because this is the first day in your journey to gaining a better understanding of how your body works and which path you should take to be a healthier You!

Let's me start this book by telling you one of my biggest secrets. But before I tell you my secret, let me give you some insight into my journey and how I came to write this book. My journey starts as a little skinny kid growing up in Baltimore, Maryland. If you know anything about the city of Baltimore, it's a tough place to grow up. The skinny kids in Baltimore either got beat-up, out-ran, out-jumped, out-muscled, bullied, and out-romanced (no girlfriends). As a skinny kid, I struggled with the same self-esteem and body image issues that overweight people struggle with. Those circumstances just didn't sit well with me and I felt that if I remained positive and focused that I could change them.

If I hadn't experienced this as a kid, I probably wouldn't have been as motivated throughout my years to improve my odds of being able to compete with the neighborhood kids....or better yet just to compete and survive in life. It's ironic that this experience revved up my will to survive and that this will continues to permeate itself even as I grow older. My life experiences in Baltimore, set in motion a lifetime committed to spiritual, physical and emotional improvement.

Fast forward 20 years. As I continued to pursue my own journey of self-improvement, I noticed people who started out with me on my journey and people who I met along the way, were suffering from debilitating health problems that were mostly preventable. In early 2000, I watched my mom transition from a happy, mobile, and caring workaholic, to a person who had to re-learn how to communicate and to move her own body after suffering from a stroke that unexpectedly stripped some of her abilities away. A stroke, that was largely preventable. I watched other friends and family suffer from other preventable diseases and health issues that nearly cost them their lives, their financial stability and their will to stay on this earth. It would be a crime and against my values for me to not share the information and knowledge that I've accumulated and used over the years to help me and my clients to reach our highest levels of physical fitness and health. This is one of the main reasons why I wrote this book.

The health and fitness information contained in this book is derived from over 20 years of life experiences, education, and training from the health and fitness industry and as a business and diversity consultant. Along with being certified with the American College of Sports Medicine (ACSM), the gold standard for personal training and with the National Academy of Sports Medicine (NASM) as a Weight Loss Specialist, I've accumulated a vast array of knowledge and experience from being a military officer, as a record breaking Division I, Defensive End (Colorado State University) and as an International Federation of Bodybuilding (IFBB) Men's Physique Pro. If it exists, I probably did it. And if I haven't, it's more than likely on my to do list. I've been a member of or trained at, almost every gym to include LA Fitness, World Gym, Gold Gym's, Planet Fitness, Lifetime Fitness and numerous Mom and Pop gyms. Health and Fitness has been my life blood ever since I did my first push-up as a kid.

THE PROBLEMS

- Obesity rates continue to climb for all races and ethnicities.[1]
- Almost 30% of the world's population over the age of 20 yrs. old are overweight.
- 200 million men are obese.
- 300 million women are obese.
- 40 million children younger than 5 years are overweight.
- Cardiovascular disease is the number 1 cause of death, globally.[2]
- 17.3 million people died of cardiovascular disease in 2008.
- 23.3 million people will die of cardiovascular disease in 2030.
- 347 million people have diabetes.
- Immigrant Asian Indian men in the U.S. have a high prevalence of coronary heart disease, non-insulin dependent diabetes, lower high density lipoprotein.[3]
- 80% of people who have diabetes or died from cardiovascular disease were in low and middle income countries.[2]
- African-Americans are nearly 1.5 times as likely to be obese compared to White adults.
- Hip fracture rates are highest in Caucasian women living in temperate climates.[5]
- African American children are more likely to be obese than their White counterparts.[10]
- 20 percent of Asian women over the age of 50 have osteoporosis and over half have low bone mass.
- Rates of deaths from heart disease and stroke are almost twice as high among African- Americans than Whites.[6]
- African Americans are twice as likely as White adults to been diagnosed with diabetes by a physician.[7]
- High rates of chronic illnesses, which in many cases are preventable, are among the biggest drivers of healthcare costs and reduce worker productivity.
- 20 percent of Caucasian women over the age of 50 have osteoporosis and over half have low bone mass.[8]
- Life expectancy for Black males was 4.7 years lower than that of White males. This difference was due to higher death rates for Black males for heart disease, homicide, cancer, stroke, and perinatal conditions.[9]
- Life expectancy for Black females was 3.3 years lower than that of White females. This difference was due to higher death rates for Black females for heart disease, cancer, diabetes, perinatal conditions, and stroke.

- Obesity rate for Caucasians increased by 11% from the period 1999-2002 to the period 2011-2012.[10]
- Obesity rate for Latinos increased by 30% from the period 1999-2002 to the period 2011-2012.[10]
- Obesity rate for Blacks increased by 21% from the period 1999-2002 to the period 2011-2012.[10]
- Individuals who weigh less than 120 pounds are at a higher risk for bone fractures.[7]
- People with a significant amount of excess body fat are at a higher risk for osteoporosis, since fat produces inflammatory factors that promote a higher rate of bone breakdown.[7]
- African-American children see twice as many calories advertised in fast food commercials as White children.[10]

THE CAUSES

- Physical inactivity
- Limited access to health and fitness information
- Conveniences such as automobiles, machinery, television, computers and other labor saving devices, produce sedentary behavior.[10]
- Social pressure to consume foods that aren't healthy.
- Lack of portion control; eating too much
- Cultural influences-" Eat everything on your plate", as learned as a child.
- Nutritional Imbalance-Eating too many carbohydrates and fats and not enough protein.
- Limited access to affordable, healthy food, especially in low income neighborhoods
- Tobacco use
- Depression
- Lack of knowledge of necessary health, nutrition and fitness information
- Limited access to parks and recreational facilities
- Cost of access to health professionals, Nutritionist, Personal Trainers, Doctors, etc., make it unaffordable to maintain a healthy lifestyle.
- Parenting with limited access to health, nutrition and fitness information.
- Body images issues which bring about low self-esteem and low confidence.
- Easy access to cheap low nutrient high calorie food from fast food restaurants.
- Limited access to supermarkets and fresh produce.
- Deceiving advertising and marketing meant to mask the true nutritional value of food.

THE ANSWERS

- Create equal access to credible health and fitness information
- Acknowledge the right of everyone to enjoy the highest attainable standards of mental and physical health
- Development and implementation of cost effective intervention strategies.
- Acknowledge existing inequities in access to affordable healthcare
- Create, implement and administer policies that create equitable health promoting environments that enable individuals, families and communities to make healthy choices and lead healthy lives.
- Build parks and trails within reasonable distances to all neighborhoods.
- Implement food portion control.
- Live in a positive supportive health focused environment, to include food, friends and family.
- Develop healthy habits.
- Perceive health and fitness as a way of life and not just an honorable mention or checkbox event.
- Learn how to cook cost saving healthy meals.
Receive periodic health physicals to include lipid and metabolic panels.
- Avoid sitting for long periods of time.
- Make in-home counseling, treatment and personal training more readily available.[3]
- Make physical activity a mandatory part of your day
- Achieve health equity.[11]
- Read this book
- Educate yourself

Change happens…...today!

Chapter 1

The Seven Rules for Fitness Success
&
Model for Change.

Control the mind...and the body will follow.

George Dorsey

This chapter represents the first step in your journey to becoming a healthier you. As in any journey, one must first plan, set goals and use directional guidance in order to reach a final destination. The rules that follow can be used as a compass to help steer your mind and body toward the achievement of your health and fitness goals. These rules were derived from my experiences and from the many people that I have met throughout my many years of being in the health and fitness industry. Please interpret these, not as strict edicts which if violated carry a stiff penalty, but as rules that can be bended and molded to fit your own life journey. My sincerest hope, is that these rules help you to achieve the success that you truly desire. So here are my rules.

7. Be unbreakable, but be flexible.

Changing your lifestyle to a healthy one, doesn't mean that you have to go "Cold Turkey". Unfortunately, the perception amongst the general public is that one must completely rearrange their lives within a very short timeframe in order to achieve their much needed fitness goals. Well I'm here to tell you that this isn't so. Improving on your current lifestyle by becoming more fitness focused, is a lifetime endeavor and it certainly doesn't happen overnight. As long as you continue to make incremental improvements, you will succeed!

- **Continue to eat your favorites foods**...in moderation. - Haven't you heard the saying, "Too much of a good thing"? In other words, anything in excess can be bad for you. Too much protein can cause dehydration. Too many vitamins can be toxic to your body. And too much exercise can cause damage to your skeletal muscle tissue (Rhabdomyolysis). By in large, people become overweight because they eat too much and move too little. So what can you do? Scale it back a little. Instead of three slices of cake. Just try 1. Instead of 4 strips of bacon. Just try 2. Instead of 3 Rum and Cokes (Cuba Libre), just have 1. Enjoy!

- **Skip your workout.** -Yes, I said it! Taking a rain check on a workout from time to time might do you some good. We all have a lot on our plates. Most of us have to work for a living and we also have to make time for family, friends, studying, socializing and everything else that makes us who we are. So, throwing in a workout, can add more stress to a person's day. Physical stress coupled with mental stress can put your body in a harmful place. Stress is stress. Like they say, Rome wasn't built in a day and neither will your body! If you're feeling like you've already had a very long and stressful day, take a day off, relax and rejuvenate...and hit it hard the next time. But don't make it a habit.

- **Don't beat yourself up**. -Guilt can be a motivator or a demotivator. Guilt can also cause anxiety and put you in a state of feeling oppressed. Self-guilt can be bad, but guilt brought on by others can be three times as bad. Guilt is brought on by a conscience understanding that you failed to live up to a certain standard. Most feel guilty because they missed a workout or ate something that was not in their nutrition plan. But that's okay, forgive yourself. Find out why you feel guilty and determine what you can do in the future to prevent this situation from happening again. Instead of feeling guilty for not completing a 45-minute workout, you can feel good for completing a more intense 25-minute workout. Instead of feeling guilty for eating 2 pieces of chocolate cake, you can feel good about not having the caramel topping that normally comes on the chocolate cake. You can always find good, even in the worst of situations.

6. Control your inner demon

The most important battle that you will ever face during your journey to become more fitness focused, is certainly not in any gym. The most important battle that you will face is the daily battle that goes on in your head. Sigmund Freud describes this as the interaction between the id, the superego and the ego. Should I eat a salad or should I eat fried chicken? Should I workout or should I watch the next episode of my favorite television show? The ego balances between the instinctual urges of the id and the values and moral standards of the superego. As we know, many times the instinctual urges of the id wins the battle. Wants, likes and needs... As I tell my clients and my friends, you have to overcome this tug of war in order to be successful to becoming a healthier you. So here are just a few steps that you can add to your tool belt to help you to win the fight!

- **Remove temptations.** -If you know that the Krispy Kreme drive-up window is on the left hand corner, right before you get home, then try to find another route home. Using alternatives to our daily patterns and habits can help to shake up things and change the normal cycle of temptations that we come across during the day. Instead of pushing your cart through the chip and cookie aisle at your favorite grocery store, take a detour to the fruit and vegetable aisle. Even if you end up at Costco or Sam's Club and you are inundated with the food pushers that they employ, it's okay to reject their advances. I do it all the time. And you know what? I feel good about myself because I could muster up the strength to just say no to food that might not be in my nutrition plan.

- **Avoid social pressures.** -Social events like cookouts, birthdays or get togethers tend to force us to eat and drink things that we know aren't healthy for us. Some of my clients feel that they need to avoid attending these events altogether for the simple fact that they know they'll feel pressure to indulge in foods that aren't in their nutrition plan. I never suggest turning yourself into a hermit to avoid the temptation of food. There are several things that you can do to help to lessen the pressure that you may feel at these events. The first method is to eat before you go. At least you know that if you're full when you get there you'll only be nibbling, instead of gorging on the food that is offered to you. Another method, is to bring your own food (BYOF). It's okay to place your 8 oz. chicken breast on the grill right next to the rack of barbecue ribs. At least you know that you're staying true to your goal of achieving a healthier you. And who knows, you'll probably set the example for others too.

- **Eat foods that make you feel full.** -Since people tend to overeat during the day because they feel hungry, eating foods that can help to increase the feeling of satiety (sə'tīətē) is recommended. Satiety is the feeling that we get when we feel full. In the early 90's, Dr. Susanna Holt of Sydney University in Australia developed the satiety index.[12] This index attempts to rank foods on their ability to make you feel full. Foods such as oatmeal that are higher in fiber and foods such as eggs and beef that are high in protein have high satiety index numbers. Foods like cake, doughnuts and candy bars have low satiety index numbers, which means that these foods won't make you feel full, at all. You can review a complete list of foods and their satiety index numbers by using the web address on this topic in the resources section at the back of this book.

5. Find out what your relationship is with food

Those who know me and those who are connected to me through social media know that I love chocolate cake. I can sit and eat an entire double fudge chocolate cake in one sitting while watching the latest Netflix movie. Then I'll feel guilty for about a week or so and I'll punish myself by working out longer or by going cold turkey. What I found out about myself is that I typically binge when I'm stressed out, so I go into the "self-soothing" mode as described in the book, "50 Ways to Soothe Yourself Without Food".[13] I also found out that I tend to be an emotional eater. I kept repeating the same cycle over and over again, so the gains that I wanted from my exercise program were not being realized. As described in this book, I had to determine what my relationship was with food and why I kept going into this cycle and how to find other ways to "soothe myself". We all tend to go through the same or similar cycles, so it is important to understand how to break these cycles, so that you can get the most out of your exercise program.

- **Turn off your "Autopilot"**-Believe it or not, our subconscious mind makes decisions for us. Both Freud and Jung agreed that unconscious thinking or cognition is the process of perception, memory, learning, thought, and language without being aware of it. The unconscious mind works without the knowledge or control of the conscious mind. Decisions are sometimes made automatically without introspection or thought. The subconscious mind acts like an internal storage center for our memories, experiences and previous thoughts. However, we can "defrag" our storage center by moving negative thoughts and memories and replacing those negative thoughts and memories with positive ones. You can change your negative habits with positive habits. For example, think of all the times that you chose to eat an unhealthy meal or snack. Eventually these negative choices become your habits. By replacing these meals or snacks with healthier foods, you can make these choices your new habits.

- **Eat consistently during the day to avoid the "bottomless pit" syndrome-** You'd be surprised how many people I talk to who tell me that they don't eat breakfast. I'd estimate that over half of thousands of people who I've spoken to about their nutrition have stated that they don't eat a meal in the morning. To fill the void, people tend to snack most of the day, eat a large lunch or a large dinner. The total calories consumed during the day tends to go over the recommended daily caloric intake, specific to their height, weight. gender and activity level. Additionally, certain metabolic processes such as muscle building and fat loss depend on a steady and consistent stream of food during the entire day and not at just one or two sittings. Be sure to eat consistently throughout the day.

- **Get help!** -If you feel that you can't go it alone, it's okay to seek help. Many companies offer Employee Assistance programs (EAP) that offer you free or low cost access to counselors, nutritionists and psychologists. Some insurance companies like Humana will even pay for your gym membership fees and Blue Cross and Medicare offer coverage for nutrition counseling. Some educational institutions like Boston University and government entities like the Northeast Health District (Georgia) offer free to low cost services.

- **Practice yoga/meditation-** These two ancient methods allow you to calm and control your body and mind. Many health facilities offer yoga or meditation classes. You can use the Yoga finder link in the resources section of this book to find a practitioner near you.

4. Live in a supportive environment.

I had a client named Jim. Jim started his workout program with as much enthusiasm and excitement as a kid headed to Disney World. Jim was told by his doctor that he had high blood pressure and was pre-diabetic. As weeks went by I started to see this enthusiasm wane. After witnessing this decline, I started asking Jim questions about his support system and his home environment so that I could find out why Jim didn't seem as committed to his workouts as he did before. After about 20 minutes of conversation, I found out why. Jim was married to a wonderful lady. However, his wife didn't quite understand how important her role was to ensuring that Jim stayed committed to achieving his physical fitness goals. When Jim would return home after his workouts, his wife who loved to cook would make Jim a five (5) course dinner to include his favorite raspberry dessert. His wife was excited for Jim and wanted to show her appreciation for his efforts by making him his favorite dishes. Jim made every attempt to explain to his wife that these type of meals were not helping him, but his wife continued. Jim's progress towards his goal of reducing his high blood pressure and lowering his glucose levels were being hampered by his wife's appreciation.

I'm sure that this scenario sounds all too familiar. In a study posted in the Journal of Consulting and Clinical Psychology, researchers found that 95% of the participants, who incorporated a social support system, completed weight loss treatment and 66% of these participants kept the weight off. For those who didn't use a support system, 76% completed the treatment and only 24% kept the weight off.[14] So here is what you can do.

- **Join social groups**-There is a vast array of social groups filled with people who are committed to achieving their physical fitness goals. Groups range from running groups, to healthy cooking groups, to bicycling groups, and counseling groups. You can get information about social groups in your local area by stopping by your local gym or fitness center or by searching the internet. Don't forget the YMCA and YWCA!

- **Join a group fitness class**-Most gyms and fitness clubs offer group exercise classes. Some of the most popular are Zumba, Spin, Water Aerobics, and boot camps. Many of the participants tend to strike up relationships with other group members and they also act to hold each other accountable.

- **Join a social media group**-Facebook, Twitter, Instagram, Meetup and other social media sites, all have groups that are dedicated to fitness. You can do a search on these sites to find a group in your local area.
- **Use a visioning board**-A visioning board is used to help you to visualize, clarify and focus on your goals. You can create a visioning board with something like a standard corkboard or you can use your tablet, computer or smartphone. Yes, there is an app for this too!

- **Educate your inner circle**-Most people within your inner circle to include your friends and family, simply don't understand their importance to helping you to achieve your physical fitness goals, unless they've experienced the same or a similar situation. It's a good idea to familiarize them with what your goals are, share why it's important to you to achieve your fitness goals and explain what they could do to help. I've helped my clients develop "behavior contracts" with themselves and also with their friends and family. This has helped to create some accountability on both sides of aisle. You can see a sample behavior contract in the appendix section of this book.

- **Celebrate the small stuff**-No matter how small you think the accomplishment is, treat it like it's one of the best days of your life. If you made it to the gym...celebrate it! If you took a walk in the park...celebrate it! If you declined the offer of pecan pie.... celebrate it! Every time an accomplishment is made use positive reinforcement to make this a habit. Using positive reinforcement strengthens the likelihood that a particular behavior will occur in the future. If I have a great workout, I'll buy a shirt that I like. If I have a full month of accomplishments, I buy myself a new pair of Jordan's. Yes, I know, another Jordan fan.

3. Find balance in your life

How many times do you think I've heard the phrase, "I just don't have time to get to the gym?" I've heard this from so many people, I lost count 15 years ago. But you know what? I understand. I'm busy too. I'm running a business, trying to spend time with family, serving my country in the Reserves, checking Facebook, looking at emails, shopping, traveling and everything else in between. I get it. But you know what they say. People will always find time to do what they really want to do. If I hid a bag with a million dollars in it, at a park or at a gym and told people that they had to be there at least 4 days each week for 45 minutes, how many people do you think would show up? Everybody. They would even bring their friends and family. Well, for a lot of people who are dealing with significant health issues, they should use the same mindset when thinking about finding time to exercise. Not like a million bucks is just sitting in a bag somewhere, but as if their lives depended on it. Let's face it. We all procrastinate from time to time. We all find time to do things that we know we shouldn't be doing. And we all find time to do things that might please us temporarily for that moment. But there is hope. You can find a happy medium and still enjoy the other things that are on your list. This is how.

- **Learn to say "No".** -My problem is I just can't say no. And when I don't say No, I tend to stack my schedule with things that I know that I shouldn't be doing. What I've learned is that it is okay to say No to things that don't help me to reach my goals and to say Yes, to things that do. If it's not helping me, then it's preventing me from reaching my goals.

- **Manage your schedule.** -How many hours are in a day? I couldn't tell you because sometimes the days just seem to blend in. Many of us have a habit of packing our schedules with events and tasks that we know is not humanly possible to complete. Managing your schedule even takes time. To help alleviate the chaos, you can make a "to do list". Categorize and prioritize everything that is on the list. Delete the tasks that don't help you to achieve your goals. You can use an online calendar like Google Calendar to help you to visualize everything that is on your plate. Once you delete the unnecessary stuff, you'll probably be surprised at how much more "extra" time you'll have in a day. Learn to take small steps when planning your schedule as well. Break big tasks down into smaller more manageable tasks.

- **Share responsibilities.** -How many people do you know that are "A" type personalities who feel that they have to do everything? They don't trust their friends, family members, co-workers or employees to complete tasks, even as simple as making coffee. I have a confession to make. I'm one of those "A" types. Well I used to be...sort of. What I've learned over the years, is that in order to get more things done, I have to trust other people by sharing responsibilities instead of hoarding them. By doing this, I freed up time on my schedule and built trust between myself and the people that I know.

- **Portion control**-. Finding balance on your plate is an essential part of finding balance in your life. Just as putting too many things on your To Do list, can cause you problems, so can putting too much food on your plate. Take a look at the portion control section in Chapter 3 for more information.

2. Know that you deserve the best in life.

Studies have shown that people who look good, radiate confidence and feel good about themselves, are happier, have better careers, get promoted, have better looking spouses, make more money and have better social interactions. In a Duke University study, researchers found that looks and confidence can drive up not only salary, but also the perception of competence.[15] It doesn't matter if you feel that you need to lose 10 to 100 lbs., you can still be beautiful, good looking and carry yourself with confidence. The state of being "good looking" is really about your self-confidence, self-awareness, the way you carry yourself and overall attitude. Trust me, I've met some people (men and women included) who would be considered "model types" but because of their lack of self-confidence, their negative outlook and poor attitude, you wouldn't want to be in the same room with them for 10 minutes. On the other hand, I've met some people who might be considered average or below average looking, but who could walk into a room and have every person's eyes pointed directly at them.

Just remember that 80% of our communication is nonverbal. What message is sent if a person walks with their head down, isn't smiling, avoids eye contact and is frowning? Does this sound like a person that you want to meet? Probably not. Don't you want the best out of life?

- **Walk with Confidence**-As I learned in the military, walk like you have a purpose. Men, ladies love a man who exudes confidence. And ladies, men love women that radiate with confidence. People could always tell that I was in the military because of how I carried myself. If you walk as tall as you can and pull your shoulders back, people will know that you're confident and you're not the one to be messed with.

- **Hold your head up high and smile**. -Unless you're reading your smartphone, looking down at the floor sends a message of uncertainty and inattentiveness. Holding your head up high sends a message that you are present, attentive and self-aware. A smile is largely interpreted in most cultures as a positive gesture or greeting. A smile sends a message of openness, friendliness and gentleness. People will normally respond well to a person who smiles.

- **Dress for the part**- What emotions do you feel when you dress up for a night on the town? Do you feel invincible, confident and ready to take on the world? Of course you do. So why not feel those same emotions during your workouts? Wearing extremely baggy clothes with holes and sweat stains, are a potential safety issue and those types of clothes certainly don't project a positive you. Wearing clothes that fit well, that are functional and that give you energy is certainly motivation to get you through your workouts. The color of your clothes can make a difference too. Colors like red, yellow and orange are claimed to give you energy. Gold and silver indicate harmony and balance. Black is a great color that actually makes you look slimmer. The fitness apparel industry has certainly caught on to this and there are many companies that offer a wide range of apparel that can fit almost every budget.

1.   Know that God has given you a gift.

Name the most precious or the most valued thing that you currently have in your possession. Some may say that their most valued possession is a vintage car, a piece of jewelry or even a family heirloom. Some will even argue that the most valued possession that anyone has, is their own body. I tend to agree. Let's face it. Name one thing that you own that can repair itself, fight off disease, jump hurdles, regulates its own temperature, make music, communicate in various ways and last but certainly not least.....create life. There should be no doubt that the human body is by far the most complex, sophisticated and unconquered thing on this earth. The human body is made up of eleven (11) different systems which perform the various functions for digestion, respiration, movement, sensing, fighting disease and a whole bunch more. Your brain controls every movement and every function in your body. It works more efficiently than any computer ever built. Even though the human body has been studied for centuries, there are still many things that doctors and scientist still do not know about the human body.

The human body is amazing! I'm sure that you've heard the phrase, "Your body is a temple...." Well that is a paraphrase of a verse pulled directly from the Bible. Some have interpreted this verse from the Bible as relating to an intangible spiritual experience, while others have related this verse to a more tangible physical experience. I interpret it as both. Regardless of your perspective, I think it's safe to say that, God has truly given us a gift, the human body. What better way to show appreciation for this gift than to maintain it, both spiritually, mentally and physically?

- **Exercise on a regular basis**-Nothing better demonstrates your appreciation for your body, by using it the way that it was meant to be used. Your body is made for movement. Being sedentary is extremely unhealthy for your body. There are a number of programs that are offered by health clubs, medical insurance companies and employee assistance programs to help to to exercise on a regular basis. There is even a program called SliverSneakers©, that offers services to more seasoned (65 and over) gym-goers. This program offers fitness classes, Program Advisors, social activities and outdoor fitness activities for over 13,000 locations throughout the United States. For more information on SilverSneakers©, please refer to the resources section of this book. Get moving!

- **Eat healthy meals**-You wouldn't pump 89 octane gas in a diesel car would you? If you want it to run correctly, you wouldn't. This same concept applies to your body. If you fuel your body with foods that are not healthy for you, your body will produce a subpar performance.

- **Get the appropriate amount of sleep**-Sleep loss or sleep disorders affect nearly 70 million people within the United States. Lack of sleep affects focus, reduces motivation to exercise, increases appetite, reduces reaction time and can cause faulty decision making. Sleep is important for specific metabolic processes such as growth and tissue repair. 7-8 hours is all it takes![18]

- **Seek emotional and mental help when needed**-Not only is physical health important, mental and emotional health is just as important. There is absolutely nothing wrong with getting assistance from a counselor or psychologist, with emotional and mental health. You're not alone. Millions of Americans are currently living with a mental disorder. Disorders range from depression all the way to eating disorders like anorexia, bulimia and binge eating. The United States is the worldwide leader, followed by Japan of deaths associated with eating disorders.[19] Due to certain cultural or religious beliefs, in-home counseling may also be available. Check my list of free to low cost mental health resources in the back of this book.

Model for Change

There are a number of behavior change models that I've used in the past such as the widely known Transtheoretical Model (TTM), Health Action Process Approach (HAPA), or the Social Cognitive Theory. Unfortunately, based on my experience of using these models, these models leave a lot to the imagination. The change model below is meant to simplify the process of change and to give the user an easily understood framework in which to create real lifestyle changes.

"Goal Achievement"

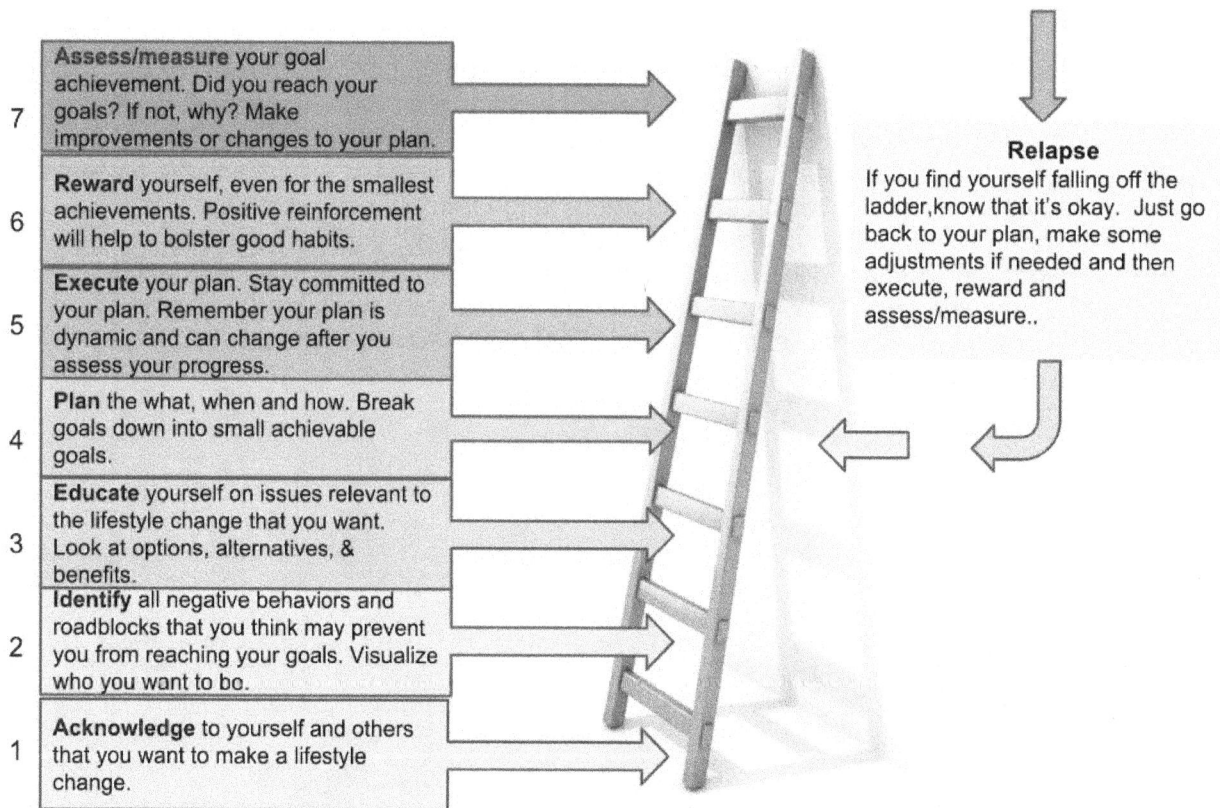

7 — **Assess/measure** your goal achievement. Did you reach your goals? If not, why? Make improvements or changes to your plan.

6 — **Reward** yourself, even for the smallest achievements. Positive reinforcement will help to bolster good habits.

5 — **Execute** your plan. Stay committed to your plan. Remember your plan is dynamic and can change after you assess your progress.

4 — **Plan** the what, when and how. Break goals down into small achievable goals.

3 — **Educate** yourself on issues relevant to the lifestyle change that you want. Look at options, alternatives, & benefits.

2 — **Identify** all negative behaviors and roadblocks that you think may prevent you from reaching your goals. Visualize who you want to be.

1 — **Acknowledge** to yourself and others that you want to make a lifestyle change.

Relapse
If you find yourself falling off the ladder, know that it's okay. Just go back to your plan, make some adjustments if needed and then execute, reward and assess/measure..

Chapter 2

The Engine
(The Digestive System)

Your success is only limited by the limitations that you set on yourself......own it.

George Dorsey

The Digestive System....why it matters.

Before you get engulfed in developing your own resistance training programs, nutrition plans and cardiorespiratory (aerobic) programs it is important that you have a basic understanding of how the systems within your body function, to give you the energy and movement to exercise. Out of all of the 11 systems that the human body contains the digestive system is the most important. The digestive system is equivalent to the engine in your car or motorcycle. Just as the engine in your vehicle converts fuel into energy, your digestive system performs in the same manner, by turning the foodstuffs that you consume, into a useable energy form, called calories. As our vehicles tend to frequently remind us, if the inner workings of our engines aren't functioning properly, neither do our vehicles. Let's face it, you wouldn't put diesel fuel in a gas powered car would you? Well some of you are, but we'll talk about that in the next chapter.

The primary purpose of the digestive system is to convert the food that we eat into energy and nutrients for the entire body. That's right, every piece of fruit, bowl of quinoa or chocolate bar has to be processed into a much smaller size to allow your body to use it as energy. You're probably asking yourself, "Why is knowing about the digestive system important to fitness?" Well, any abnormality or problem with any component of the digestive system could have a negative impact on your performance and overall health. It is important for you to understand the components of the digestive system and the most frequently experienced health problems that negatively affect them. Any slight problem with any of these components could negatively impact how your body processes the food that you eat which ultimately affects your ability to produce movement, and the ability of your body to grow and repair itself.

For example, I had a client named Kim. Kim frequently complained about feelings of heartburn and indigestion. As we started to progress to more advanced physical activities in her workout plan, Kim's performance started to decline. Kim just passed off these feelings as a simple case of heartburn. I would frequently see Kim take large amounts of antacid medicine. I finally had to inform Kim that it was best that she discontinue her exercise program until she figured out what was causing her so much discomfort. After I questioned Kim about the foods that she was eating, I learned that Kim loved pickled food. Kim frequently ate pickled meat and pickled eggs and has been doing so for quite some time. I explained to Kim that the ingestion of large amounts of pickled foods could cause a peptic ulcer to occur in the lining of the stomach or upper small intestine, or it could also lead to more serious issues like stomach cancer. This information shocked Kim enough for her to see a doctor. Kim was eventually diagnosed with gastritis which is an inflammation of the stomach lining. Kim eventually stopped eating pickled foods and the frequent discomfort that she felt subsided.

The digestive system consists of the following components;

- Mouth (oral cavity)
- Teeth
- Esophagus
- Stomach
- Small intestine
- Large intestine (rectum)
- Liver
- Pancreas
- Gall Bladder

Whether it's a Big Mac with cheese or a quinoa salad, the process of digestion is the same for all foods. However, not all parts of your meal end up at the same place at the same time. Some parts of your food get digested faster, while other parts of your meal get digested slower. The chart below gives you specific timeframes for the time it takes your body to digest food. In general, it takes 40 hours for food to pass from your mouth before it is expelled from your body.

The Digestive System

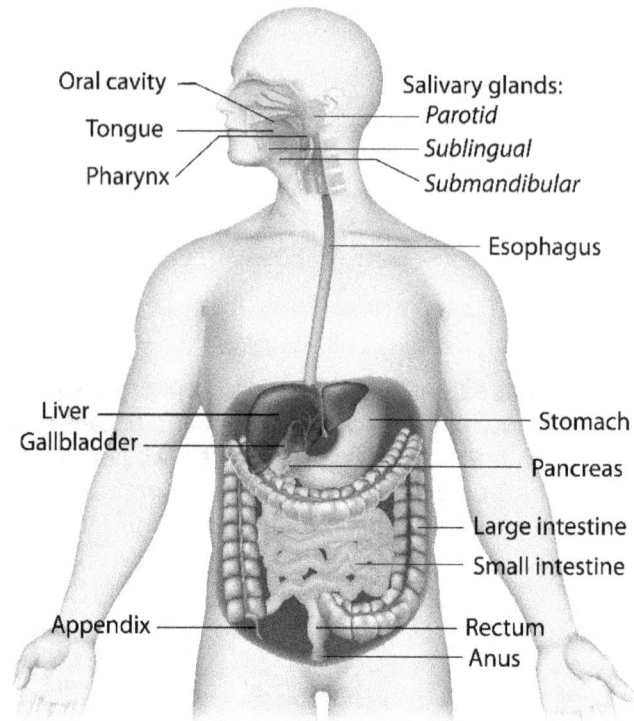

Oral cavity

Tongue

Pharynx

Salivary glands:
Parotid
Sublingual
Submandibular

Esophagus

Liver

Gallbladder

Stomach

Pancreas

Large intestine

Small intestine

Appendix

Rectum

Anus

Digestion-Food processing times[20]	
50% of stomach contents are emptied	2.5 to 3 hours
Total emptying of the stomach	4 to 5 hours
50% emptying of the small intestine	2.5 to 3 hours
Transit through the colon	30 to 40 hours

The food we eat travels through six main parts of the body; which are called the alimentary canal 1) Mouth 2) Pharynx 3) Esophagus 4) Stomach 5) Small intestine 6) Large intestine.

Just like in a car's engine, each stage of the fuel conversion process serves different and very important functions.

Mouth (Oral Cavity)

Have you ever found your mouth watering while thinking about your favorite foods? Well this is your brain telling your mouth to release saliva which contains enzymes that are essential for the digestion process. When the food we eat enters the mouth our body starts to immediately work to breakdown the food. Our mouth contains various things such as teeth, glands and tongue that start the process of breaking down the food we eat for further processing.

Other than being called a "grill", your teeth play a very important role in digestion. (That was a joke by the way.) Humans get two sets of teeth during a lifetime. Your teeth perform different functions depending on their location and shape.

The four teeth located in the front of your mouth called incisors are used for biting into and cutting food. The two fang like teeth directly next to your incisors are called canines (Yes just like a dog.) and are used for grasping and tearing. As we move further towards the rear of the mouth, the next four teeth after your canines are called premolars. These teeth are flatter than your canines and are used for grinding. Moving all the way to the rear of your mouth, the next six teeth are called molars. Your molars are broader than your premolars and are used to prepare your food for swallowing, by grinding and mixing your food.

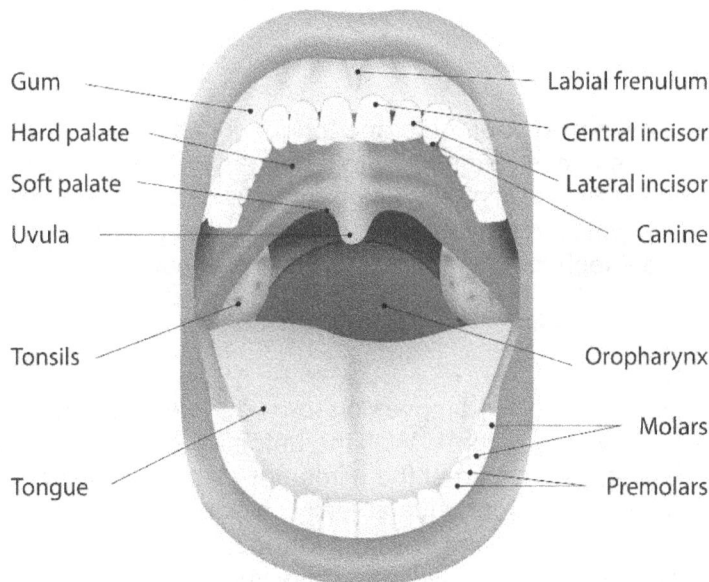

The act of chewing breaks down food into smaller particles for easier digestion. Chewing actually increases blood flow to the mouth and to the head. The taste buds on your tongue stimulate saliva production. The saliva from your salivary glands helps to prepare the food (bolus-a small round mass of food.) you just ate for digestion and also begins the breakdown of carbohydrates.

As you can see, your teeth play a significant role in the digestion process. Each group of teeth have very distinct functions which are important to the digestion process. Poor oral hygiene, eating lots of sugary or processed foods and using tobacco products can damage your teeth and gums. Worldwide, 9 out of 10 people over 40 years of age have some form of periodontal disease.[21] Periodontal disease can cause heart disease, because bacteria from periodontal disease can enter the bloodstream, contributing to clot formation in coronary arteries. It is extremely important for you to take care of your teeth and gums by brushing and flossing regularly.

The role of Saliva
- Dissolves & lubricates food
- Contains an enzyme that initiatives chemical digestion of carbohydrates
- Frees the mouth and teeth of food
- Produces the sensation of thirst to prevent dehydration

Pharynx

Once your food moves past your teeth and tongue it heads downward into the pharynx. The pharynx is almost like a foyer in a house. Just as a foyer might open up to different rooms like the hallway, kitchen, dining room or den, the pharynx has openings to the nasal cavity, oral cavity, the larynx and esophagus. For purposes of this book, we will only talk about the esophagus as the next step in our journey.

Esophagus

Once past the pharynx, your food moves on toward the esophagus. I'm sure you've heard of the saying, "Down the hatch!". Well the hatch is just another name for the esophagus. The esophagus is a part of the alimentary canal and is about 10 inches long and a ½ inch in diameter. The esophagus actually carries food through three sections of your body; your neck; your thorax and down to your abdomen. The esophagus curves 1 inch slightly to the left of your body's midline. Have you ever seen a snake eat an animal that is much bigger than the snake? If so, you may have seen the body of the snake grow and take on the shape of the animal that it is eating. Your esophagus acts in a similar way in that it "distends" or stretches to accommodate the size of the food or bolus that is coming down the hatch. The esophagus is actually made up of muscles which act to push the bolus downward in a movement called, "peristalsis". Eventually your food will make its way down to your stomach.

The esophagus is prone to damage when the sphincter between the esophagus and the stomach malfunctions and allows stomach content saturated with hydrochloric acid to back up into the esophagus. A severe version of this is called gastroesophageal reflux disease or GERD.[21] People who suffer from this condition should limit their consumption of foods like tomatoes or coffee.

Stomach

Compared to the other parts of the body that we just discussed, the stomach is fairly large with a length of 1 foot and the width of six inches. The stomach of a human can normally hold about one quart of food, but can distend to hold as much as four quarts or about 20 times its volume when empty. Only a few nutrients are absorbed into the bloodstream from the stomach, because the stomach lining cannot absorb most nutrients. However, the lining's mucus secreting cells can absorb water, alcohol, and aspirin. These substances are actually absorbed in the body much faster than other substances that we might consume. The stomach is actually made up of folds called "rugae". When the stomach starts to reach its capacity the rugae expand to enlarge the stomach. Once the food is inside your stomach, various chemical and mechanical processes take place in which gastric juices are released into the stomach. The stomach contains three types of gastric glands; 1) Cardiac, 2) Pyloric, and 3) Fundic. These gastric juices reduce the food into a thick semiliquid mass called "chyme". This chyme will eventually find its way into the small intestine within 1 to 4 hours of when the food was consumed.

The food that we eat in whole or in part will follow the entire digestive tract starting from the mouth to the anus. As food follows the digestive tract or alimentary canal, as it is technically called, digestive enzymes continue to work to break down the food that you just ate.

Peristalsis-is a series of muscle contractions that occur automatically in the digestive tract.

Rugae- are ridges or folds in the lining of stomach. As the stomach fills and then stretches, the rugae smooths out.

Enzyme-a protein that acts to breakdown food. Enzymes perform at their peak at normal body temperature 98.6 degrees F.

Sphincter-a muscle that surrounds and controls an opening in the body.

Small Intestine

Believe it or not, this is where most of the action happens. The small intestine is the place where most digestion takes place, not in your stomach. The small intestine is approximately 20 feet long. The small intestine contains almost 2,700 square feet of surface area, about the size of a good sized house, for absorbing nutrients into the bloodstream.[23] This is also the place where your body absorbs most of the macronutrients such as carbohydrates, fats and proteins and micronutrients such as vitamins and minerals, into the bloodstream.   The small intestine is divided into three regions, 1) Duodenum, 2) Jejunum 3) Ileum

Food that is not absorbed into the bloodstream is passed out from the alimentary canal by a process called egestion (egestion-The act or process of discharging undigested or waste material from a cell or organism). Fat, however is not absorbed directly into the bloodstream. Fats go through lymphatic vessels before fat is delivered to general circulation.

Large Intestine

Just think of the large intestine as a 5-foot long funnel. The large intestine is about 3 inches wide at the top of the funnel and decreases in width as you move down the length of it. Chyme (Chyme-the semifluid mass of partly digested food expelled by the stomach into the duodenum) from the small intestine moves its way down the entire length of the large intestine. The large intestine is broken down into 5 regions: Cecum----Vermiform appendix-----Ascending colon----Transverse colon--- Descending colon----Sigmoid colon----Rectum---- Anus.[24]

Compared to the small intestine, the large intestine is pretty boring. Most of the body's water absorption occurs in the large intestine. The large intestine has no digestive function and only secretes mucus. The large intestine and more specifically the end of the large intestine, truly represents the end of the journey for the food that you ate only 40 hours ago.

As you can tell, the intestines play a major role in the digestion process. Your body gets most of its nutrients from the work that the intestines perform. Inflammatory diseases like Crohn's disease causes inflammation and ulcers in the intestinal wall. Some intestinal diseases and disorders can be prevented by eating a well-balanced diet.

The pancreas, liver and gallbladder, although not directly a part of the digestive system, play vital roles in the digestive process.

Pancreas

The pancreas plays two complementary but very important roles in the digestive process. The first role is that of an endocrine gland, by secreting much needed hormones like insulin and glucagen which help to regulate blood sugar. The second role is that of an exocrine gland, by secreting pancreatic juices that contain enzymes which can breakdown all types of food, making these juices most important to the digestive process.

Things such as gallstones, heavy consumption of alcohol, cigarette smoking, high triglycerides (high cholesterol), high blood sugar, obesity, surgery, metabolic disorders and medications can cause pancreatitis and/or diabetes (Type 2). Heavy consumption of alcohol and gallstones account for over 80% of all cases of pancreatitis in the United States.[25] This disease can cause pain in the upper abdomen which can also be felt in the back. Weight loss can occur due to the pancreas not releasing enough enzymes to break the food down which prevents the body from absorbing the food.

In 2012, over 29 million Americans had diabetes.[26] In Type 2 diabetes, your body becomes insulin resistant and eventually the human body can no longer make enough insulin to manage blood glucose levels within a normal range. Diabetes may also develop if the insulin producing cells of the pancreas are damaged.

As a preventative measure, those with high cholesterol or high blood glucose should develop nutrition and exercise programs which are aimed at reducing body fat and increasing cardiorespiratory fitness.

Liver

The liver of a human is the largest gland in the human body. The liver is looked upon as a workaholic gland that is able to multitask and juggle very important responsibilities. Running down the list of responsibilities, the liver produces blood plasma proteins to ward against disease, heparin which is a blood anticoagulant that prevents clotting, and bile that assist in fat digestion and removal of excess cholesterol from the blood. The liver stores vitamins, minerals and glucose, in the form of glycogen. Without the liver conversion and utilization of fats, carbohydrates and proteins would not be possible.[27] The liver also acts as a filter by removing non-functioning red blood cells, toxins and waste products from amino acid breakdown.
Diseases such as hepatitis, cirrhosis and gallstones (high cholesterol) can damage the liver which ultimately affect liver performance.

Gallbladder

The gallbladder is nestled directly under the liver. This organ stores bile produced by the liver, to be released later to help the human body to digest fats. The gallbladder is not an essential organ and can be removed without any known side effects. Gallstones can develop in the gallbladder which can cause pain, nausea or inflammation. Gallbladder cancer, although rare, can develop in the tissues of the gallbladder from malignant cancer cells.

Why is knowing your body type important?

Knowing your body type can help you to better understand how your body may respond to your weight loss or weight gain efforts. Your body type can also be an indicator of your potential level of athletic performance. Over 70 years ago psychologist William Sheldon attempted to categorize body shapes to indicate temperament, intelligence, moral character and future achievement. The process that Sheldon used is called "somatotyping". Most, if not all of his work related to the psychological aspect of somatotyping has been discredited. However, the physiological aspect of the categories that he developed are still in use to this day. Sheldon developed three main body types, Ectomorph, Mesomorph and Endomorph. No person fits neatly into one of these categories. A person may share characteristics of more than one of these categories.

All too often I hear people complain that their exercise regimen fails to produce results. The thin claim to not be able to gain weight and those who have identified themselves as "overweight", claim to not be able to lose any weight. There is some truth to their concerns. However, their problems largely lie in the way that they develop and carry out their nutrition and physical fitness strategies and not necessarily in their body type. Here are the reasons why.

Ectomorph

I'm sure that you've met people in your life that can eat just about anything and never gain any weight. During my years in health and fitness, I've found that people who boast about not being able to gain weight even after gorging themselves with food for years, typically fall into the Ectomorph body type. The Ectomorph is able to metabolize substrates like carbohydrates, fats and proteins a lot faster than their somatotype brothers and sisters. However, there are some issues that Ectomorphs need to be aware of. Ectomorph's usually have weak abdominal muscles which result in posture issues like kyphosis, lordosis or scoliosis.

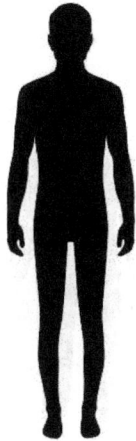

Ectomorph

Ectomorph's thyroids are generally hyperactive which increase their calorie burning capacity. In order to improve on these issues, Ectomorphs must attempt to strengthen their muscle mass through a well thought out resistance training program. Ectomorphs should also increase their caloric intake throughout the day in order to increase their weight and build muscle mass. I'm also considered an Ectomorph. As a child and teenager, I was always considered skinny. When my grandparents would come visit me or I visited them they would always provide me with cod liver oil and slim-sized Toughskin pants. According to my grandmother, the cod liver oil was meant to put some "meat" on my bones and the pants were to cover my extremely slim figure. Love 'em! However, as I aged I learned that in order to increase my weight I had to increase my daily caloric intake. I also had to develop a workout plan that was aimed at increasing my muscle mass.

Athletes who are Ectomorphs tend to compete in sports like swimming, marathon running, cycling, basketball, tennis, baseball (some positions) or gymnastics.

Mesomorph

You can always tell who is a Mesomorph by the size of their wrists, calves and shoulders. Mesomorphs tend to have larger bone structure and waist lines as compared to their somatotype brothers and sisters. Men mostly fall into this category because Mesomorphs tend to have high testosterone levels. Some books even state that men fall into this category due to millions of years of natural selection. During this time, men needed powerful bodies in order to survive and produce. However, women can be Mesomorphs as well. Mesomorphs have higher than average muscle mass. Becoming overweight is not an issue with this group if they stay active. Nutrition and physical fitness programs should be developed to help to maintain muscle mass, increase flexibility and to increase cardiorespiratory fitness.

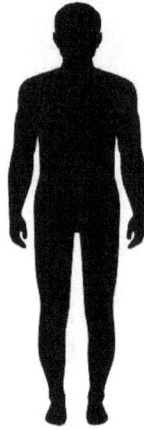

Mesomorph

You'll find Mesomorphs in mostly any sort of athletic competition. Football, hockey, and rugby are sports that are usually filled with Mesomorphs.

Endomorph

Endomorphs tend to carry a little bit more body fat than Mesomorphs and certainly more than Ectomorphs. Endomorphs look softer and normally do not have any muscular tone. This group is usually characterized as being "pear" shaped. This category is mostly claimed by women for the simple fact that women are built for child rearing and need additional body fat to carry and to feed their babies. The thyroids of Endomorphs are the least active compared to their somatotype comparators. This means that their metabolism is slower and they don't need to eat a lot in order to maintain their weight.

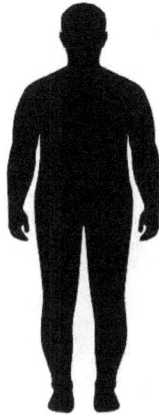

Endomorph

Endomorphs should develop a nutrition plan and physical activity plan aimed at reducing body fat and increasing muscle mass through a balanced resistance training and cardiorespiratory program. Increasing protein intake has also been an effective way to complement these strategies.

Endomorphs are inclined to compete in powerlifting and football, where explosive movements are needed. Which body type are you?

Differences in body fat distribution

Believe it or not, males and females store body fat in different places throughout their bodies. There are specific genetic reasons as to why this occurs, which will be explained in the sections that follow. There are two body fat distribution patterns which are called Gynoid for women and Android for men. However, men or women could potentially fall into either category.

Gynoid

Females on average tend to carry more body fat than men for the simple fact that women are capable of bearing children. Women use this additional body fat as energy reserves especially during the last two trimesters of pregnancy. Fat is accumulated in 9 main areas of the body to include the buttocks, lower back, hips, between the thighs, around the naval, pubis, knees, rear of the upper arm, and breasts.[28]
Women in different localities also carry body fat in different areas of the body. For example, in hot countries, body fat is highly concentrated in the buttocks (African/South American) and on the hips for women in the Mediterranean and around the navel for women in Asia. For health reasons, women should always strive to maintain a certain

amount of body fat. Extremely low body fat in women tend to produce problems with menstruation, ovulation and hormone production.[28]

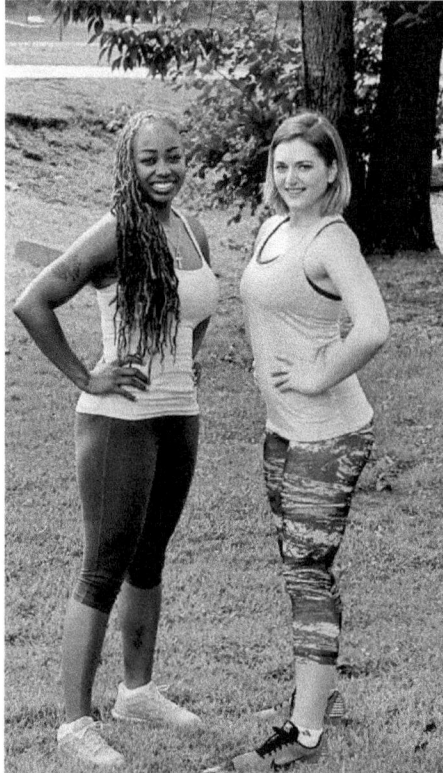

For women who are concerned about too much "Junk in the trunk...it's not your fault.

Women whose ancestors originate from warmer parts of the world such as below the equator, tend to carry more body fat in their buttocks and hips than their northern sisters. Sometimes this accumulated fat in the buttocks and hips, as an energy reserve, clumbs between the skin and the muscle, when more energy (calories) are consumed than used. This fat is spread in clusters and is walled off by fibrous connective tissue. On the surface of the skin around the buttock and hip areas you may see slight depressions in the skin which are sometimes affectionately called, "cottage cheese". This visual effect is caused by inelastic fibrous tracts which like cables, attach the envelope of the muscles to the deep surface of the skin at the depressions with the fatty tissue bulging in between. The effects look much the same as your comforter on your bed. As the fat reserves increase the fat that is contained in this net like material becomes compressed, along with your blood vessels and lymphatics, making it harder for your body to remove the excess fatty acids. At times, even dieting or extensive training may not reduce these areas.[28] Women who want to lose fat in these areas should consider adjusting their macronutrient percentages (%fats vs. %carbohydrates vs %protein) and increasing the intensity of their aerobic (cardiorespiratory) and anaerobic activities.

Android

No, I'm not referring to the Android system for your Smartphone or an Android robot. Android fat distribution is characterized by fat accumulation around the midsection and upper body. As the graphic shows, in Android fat distribution, fat accumulates in five main areas including chest, abdomen, thighs, lower back and upper buttocks. This fat accumulation distribution is also called "central obesity" or is affectionately known as "heart attack fat" by many men that I meet during my travels. Although women can have this pattern of body fat distribution, this pattern is more associated with men and can be a significant area of concern. So why is this fat accumulation pattern called "heart attack fat"? It's called this because fat mostly accumulates in the midsection, in and around vital organs like your heart, liver, kidneys and lungs.

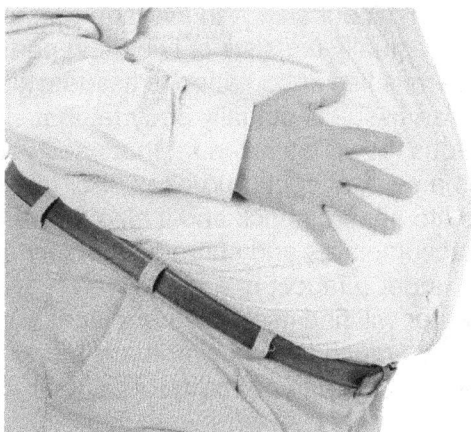

Android fat pattern can cause a significant risk to your health. Cardiovascular disease, diabetes and other metabolic diseases are highly associated with this type of fat accumulation pattern.

If you are concerned about your risk for health issues due to central obesity, there is a quick and sure way to check your risk. The hip-to waist ratio is used by health professionals to determine risk. To measure, both women and men must measure their waists right above the belly button (iliac crest) and measure their hips at the widest point. For males a waist to hip ratio of .90 or higher is an indicator of an increased risk for health issues. For females, a waist to hip ratio of .85 or higher is an indicator of an increased risk for health issues.

Example:
Male waist measurement= 38 inches, Hips= 50 inches,

38/50=.**76**. .**76** is less than .90, so this male has a low risk for health issues associated with central obesity.

Weight loss tip-Dieting alone will result in a loss of 69% body fat and 31% muscle mass for every pound lost. With the proper resistance training, one can achieve a weight loss consisting of 97% fat and only 3% muscle for every pound lost. Our aging population should pay particular attention to these numbers since muscle wasting (sarcopenia) and bone density(osteoporosis) issues mainly affect this group. Losing weight without incorporating a good resistance training program to fight these effects is like burning a candle at both ends. Resistance training along with the proper nutrition plan, can help to build muscle and increase bone density even while losing weight.

Types of body fat

Subcutaneous fat

What is your body's largest organ? Your skin. An average person has a skin surface of 17 to 20 square feet.[27] Your skin actually consists of two main parts; the dermis and epidermis. Directly under the epidermis lies subcutaneous tissue which consists of areolar and adipose tissue. Adipose tissue is actually body fat that sits directly under the skin, hence the name "subcutaneous fat". This is the fat that uses your skin as camouflage. This fat actually has a several good purposes. For one, subcutaneous fat acts as a cushion to help the body to absorb shock and it also acts as insulation, by preventing heat loss. Excess fat accumulates and spreads in a very specific way. Just as if you were to put an empty glass under a faucet of running water, eventually the glass will become full and the excess water will find itself in other places. Your skin or the subcutaneous tissue can only hold so much fat and eventually the excess fat will find its way through almost every nook and cranny in your body. This is a good segway into our next topic, visceral fat.

Visceral fat

Visceral fat is the fat that causes the most concern. Visceral fat can find its way in and around your organs and blood vessels. Excess visceral fat is most associated with such health issues as cardiovascular disease, high blood pressure, and insulin resistance. Men are especially susceptible to these diseases because of the high visceral fat accumulation in the abdominal area. Men with excessively large abdomens should be concerned about visceral body fat and the risk associated with it.

Heard of Skinny Fat?

Skinny Fat is the more common term for metabolically obese normal weight. This condition is characterized by high body fat and normal body weight. In a study published in the Journal of the American Medical Association, nearly 1 out of every 4 skinny people were pre-diabetic and were metabolically obese. This study also showed that adults who were normal weight at the time of incident diabetes had a higher mortality than adults who were overweight or obese.[29] So what can you do? For starters, get your body fat checked. Various methods to measure your body fat are listed later on in this book. You should also check the body fat % charts in this book to see if in fact your body fat percentage is not within a normal range. You can also develop a resistance training program, cardiorespiratory (aerobic) program and nutrition plan to help you to lose body fat and gain muscle.

	Body Fat Norms Ages 18-25		Body Fat Norms Ages 26-35[30]	
	Men (% fat)	Women (% fat)	Men (% fat)	Women (% fat)
Excellent	3-7	9-17	4-10	7-16
Good	8-10	18-19	11-13	18-20
Above Average	11-12	20-21	14-16	21-22
Average	13-15	22-23	17-19	23-25
Below Average	16-18	24-26	20-22	26-28
Poor	19-21	27-30	23-26	29-32
Very Poor	23-35	32-43	27-38	34-46

	Body Fat Norms Ages 36-45		Body Fat Norms Ages 46-55	
	Men (% fat)	Women (% fat)	Men (% fat)	Women (% fat)
Excellent	5-13	9-18	8-16	12-21
Good	15-17	19-22	17-19	23-25
Above Average	18-20	23-25	20-22	26-28
Average	21-22	26-28	23-24	29-30
Below Average	23-25	29-31	25-27	31-33
Poor	26-28	32-35	28-30	34-37
Very Poor	29-39	37-47	31-40	39-50

| | Body Fat Norms Ages 56-65 | | Body Fat Norms Ages over 65 | |
	Men (% fat)	Women (% fat)	Men (% fat)	Women (% fat)
Excellent	11-17	12-22	12-18	11-20
Good	19-21	24-26	19-20	22-25
Above Average	22-23	27-29	21-22	26-28
Average	24-25	30-32	23-24	29-31
Below Average	26-27	33-35	25-26	32-34
Poor	28-29	36-38	27-29	35-37
Very Poor	31-40	39-49	30-39	38-45

Visceral fat can actually make you fatter....

Did you know that body fat can secrete hormones which can make you gain more weight? Body fat can act just like an endocrine (gland) organ in your body, by secreting hormones like leptin, interleukin-6, and adiponectin. These hormones affect regulation of satiety (feeling full), carbohydrate and lipid metabolism and insulin sensitivity. Leptin, sometimes called the "satiety hormone," is a hormone made by adipose cells (fat tissue) that helps to regulate energy balance by inhibiting hunger. Leptin inhibits hunger and another hormone ghrelin often called the "hunger hormone", increases hunger. Both hormones act on receptors in the arcuate nucleus of the hypothalamus to regulate appetite in order to achieve energy homeostasis. As you gain weight your sensitivity to leptin decreases, resulting in an inability to detect satiety (fullness) despite high energy stores. Adiponectin enhances your muscle's ability to use carbohydrates for energy, boosts your metabolism, increases the rate in which your body breaks down fat, and curbs your appetite. Obese individuals have been found to have lower levels of adiponectin than their non-obese counterparts. Those with a high concentration of abdominal body fat (central obesity) are highly susceptible to having lower levels of adiponectin. Not to say that everyone shouldn't be concerned with this issue, but African Americans should be particularly focused on this issue. A study in the Journal of Applied Physiology showed that the skeletal muscle of African-Americans have a reduced ability to oxidize fatty acid as compared to their Caucasian counterparts. Blacks were shown to have a reduced level of AMPK (adenosine monophosphate-activated protein kinase) activation and decreased adiponectin which may contribute to a predisposition to weight gain and insulin resistance.[31] In layman's terms AMPK and adiponectin allows your body to burn body fat. Reduced levels of these two hormones limits your body's ability to burn excess body fat. As our body fat increases the level of adiponectin in our body decreases.

Interleukin-6 is another hormone that is secreted from body fat (adipose tissue). Interleukin-6 levels are elevated with obesity and diabetes and are negatively correlated to insulin stimulated glucose disposal. Simply put, the more body fat that is gained, increases the levels of Interleukin-6 which in turn inhibits your body's ability to metabolize glucose.

So what can you do to reverse this cycle? You can maximize the levels of these hormones by exercising on a daily basis and by reducing body fat, especially abdominal body fat. Some people have found success by replacing carbohydrates in their diets with monounsaturated fats (olives, avocados, etc). But before you make any dietary changes, you may want to consult with a certified nutritionist.

How does our body burn body fat and substrates like carbohydrates, fats and proteins?

In order for your body to move, it must have energy. Your body gets its energy by using chemical processes to convert foodstuffs like carbohydrates, fats, and proteins into a biologically usable form of energy.

All energy comes from the sun. The process starts with plants that use light energy from the sun to form carbohydrates, fats and proteins. We as humans, then eat plants and other animals to get the energy that we need to maintain cellular activities. Our muscles convert chemical energy obtained from carbohydrates, fats or proteins into mechanical energy to perform movement. This process is called bioergenetics.[32]

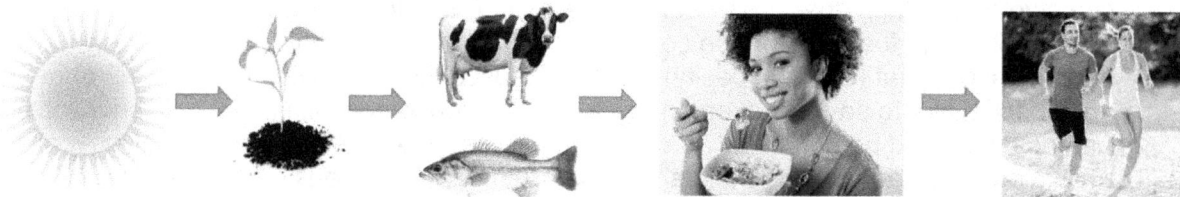

Although there are quite a few important pieces to the puzzle of bioergentics, one of the most important are enzymes. Enzymes, which are molecules that start or accelerate chemical processes help your body to metabolize fats, carbohydrates and proteins. Enzymes work best at a normal body temperature of 98.6 degrees Fahrenheit. You may ask why are enzymes important? Along with helping to regulate the speed that your body metabolizes substrates, the presence of enzymes in your blood can indicate specific health problems. When tissues within your body become diseased, dead tissues release enzymes. For example, an elevated amount of the enzyme "creatine kinase" found in the blood, can be an indicator of a heart attack (myocardial infarction) or muscular dystrophy. Other examples are listed in the table below.[32]

Enzyme	Indicator of
Lactate dehydrogenase	Myocardial infarction (heart attack)
Alkaline Phosphatase	Carcinoma of bone (cancer). Paget's disease, obstructive jaundice
Amylase	Pancreatitis, perforated peptic ulcer
Aldolase	Muscular dystrophy

How does my body use the food that I eat for energy? *Energy Systems*

Now that you are more familiar with how your body digests the food that you eat, I'm sure you are wondering how your body uses this food for energy. Your body has three systems or process which convert your food into chemical energy and then into mechanical energy for movement. The three systems are ;1) ATP-CP Phosphagen System (Anaerobic); 2) Anaerobic Glycolysis/Lactic Acid system; 3) Oxidative/Aerobic System.[32]

Before I go into detail about how these systems work to produce energy, there a few basic, but fundamental concepts that you must know. ATP or Adenosine Triphosphate provides energy for every biological process. Just think of ATP as fuel for your body, just like gas is fuel for a car. Your body is unable to move without ATP. Your body has a very small gas tank and can only store small amounts of ATP. So your body has to create its own fuel as ATP for sustained movement. It's kind of like having your own gas station at your disposal.

ATP-CP Phosphagen System (Anaerobic-without oxygen)

You just checked your map app on your smartphone and found out that your destination can be reached by walking 20 minutes. It's a nice day so you head off. But you look at your watch and find that you are running short of time, so your walk turns into a sprint. So you're off to the races! Well kind of. Your body has no fuel. But you're in luck, the ATP-CP Phosphagen System is the quickest way for your body to create ATP for fuel. What is amazing about this system is that it uses no oxygen (anaerobic) and uses no substrates like, carbohydrates, fats or protein. However, there are limitations to this system. ATP is created from Creatine Phosphate (creatine phosphate or phosphocreatine is synthesized in the liver and transported to muscle cells via the bloodstream. It is formed from parts from three amino acids.), which is stored in your muscles. Your muscles can only store a limited amount of creatine phosphate, so many athletes take creatine monohydrate to increase the stores of muscle creatine phosphate or phosphocreatine. The energy that is produced by this system can only sustain all-out movement for no more than 10 seconds.[32]

This particular energy system is mainly used by athletes who powerlift, play football or basketball, sprint or high jump. Since this system does not use carbohydrates, fats or protein for energy, it is not the best system to use for weight loss.

Glycolysis/Lactic Acid System

Just as you'd expect your map app was wrong and your destination is longer than you expected. So now your sprint is turning into a steady paced run. However, you need more energy. Remember those carbohydrates that you ate? Well now your body needs them. The glycolysis/lactic acid system (glycolysis-breakdown of glucose.) breaks down the carbohydrates (glucose-also known as "blood sugar" is a simple sugar or monosaccharide found in foods or in your body. Glucose is sometimes called dextrose.) you ate and/or the glycogen that is stored in your muscle fibers into pyruvic acid or lactic acid. This system will give your body enough energy to last 1-3 minutes or enough to run a distance of 400-800 meters.[32]

Because our bodies can only store a limited amount of glycogen, athletic performance can be hampered when glycogen stores are depleted. However, there is a way to increase the amount of glycogen stores through a process called supercompensation. This process involves the usage of strenuous exercise to exhaust the existing glycogen stored in the muscles. Then a fat/protein diet is consumed for three days while continuing to train. For the final step, a high carbohydrate diet (90% carbohydrates) is consumed for three days while ceasing any physical activity. Some studies have found that the best time to attempt to increase glycogen stores is to ingest carbohydrates immediately after exercise because there is an increase in the muscle cell's permeability to glucose, an increase in glycogen synthase activity and an increase in the muscle's sensitivity to insulin. Using either of these processes to increase glycogen stores is not recommended for use in weight loss strategies. Athletes trying to maximize their performance should take steps to ensure the proper consumption of carbohydrates.

Oxidative/Aerobic System

Our last but certainly not least energy system is the most complicated. This system is sometimes called oxidative phosphorylation and is a 3 stage process. This process uses oxygen and creates energy by breaking down carbohydrates, fats and proteins to create ATP. This system is only limited by the amount of oxygen and calories available to the body for use. This system is used mainly by individuals involved in running for distances longer than 400 meters or who perform physical activity for longer than 4 minutes. [32] For those concerned about weight loss, this is the process that has shown to breakdown (use) more carbohydrates, fats and proteins than any other energy system. Physical activity performed for extended periods of time while raising the heart rate to a specific beat per minute is a sure way to lose weight. There is more information on developing cardiorespiratory exercise programs later in this book.

Chapter 3

The Fuel
(Nutrition)

Learn to eat for a purpose and not so much for pleasure.

George Dorsey

The secret is out! There is a new miracle that just hit the health and fitness industry. This miracle is virtually guaranteed to help you to lose weight, gain muscle and reduce your risk for certain diseases. Are you interested? Now for the secret unveiling. Drum roll please……… The miracle is…ta da….a healthy diet. Proper nutrition is the holy grail of health and fitness. There is no way around it. Without it, our bodies don't function the way that they were meant to. Without it, reaching our fitness goals will absolutely be impossible.

Over the last 40 years several government, private and not for profit organizations have published their versions of nutritional recommendations in an effort to arm individuals with information to help them to make healthy food choices. Starting in 1980, the US Department of Health and Human Services (HHS) and the US Department of Agriculture published the Dietary Guidelines for Americans, which are updated every 5 years. The Institute of Medicine (IOM) also published their version of dietary recommendations in 2002. The IOM replaced the widely known terms "recommended daily allowance" (RDA) with "Dietary Reference Intakes" (DRI) starting in the mid 90's. Even the American Heart Association has jumped into the fray by publishing their "Diet and Lifestyle Recommendations". As you can see there are a number of health related organizations and individuals who all have their own opinion and ideas about what you should and what you shouldn't be eating. So how are you supposed to make sense of it all?

As we discussed in Chapter 1, think of the food that you eat as energy. Too little energy and our bodies respond with subpar performance. Too much energy and we become overweight or obese. As the first rule of thermodynamics states, energy can be transformed from one form to the other, but cannot be created or destroyed. In everyday jargon, this just means that the food (energy) that we eat, if not fully used, will transform into stored energy, like excess body fat.

A March 2000 study in the New England Journal says the average annual weight gain in adults between the ages of 25-44 is 3.4 percent for men and 5.2 percent for women.[33] For a man who normally weighs 180 lbs., this equates to over 6 lbs. of weight gain per year. For a woman who normally weighs 130 lbs., this equals to almost 7 lbs. of weight gain per year.   As you can see, after only a few years of this type of weight gain, you could easily become overweight or obese.

Before we jump deep into the topic of nutrition, let's tackle a few basic principles. The first principle is related to calories and weight loss. In short, a person must burn 3,500 calories for 1 lb. of weight loss. This means that for someone to lose 20 lbs., they must burn at least 70,000 calories. Now I know that this sounds like a lot, but it can be done and I'll show you how. It's all about the numbers.

The second principle has to do with the total amount of energy (calories) that our bodies need to maintain its current weight, to lose weight or to gain weight. There are several measures that are used to determine how many calories we should eat on a daily basis.

Those measures are Basal Energy Requirement also called Basal Metabolic Rate (BMR), Resting Metabolic Rate (RMR) and Total Daily Energy Expenditure (TDEE). The total number of calories that we need to maintain our current weight, while laying on our backs (supine), in a thermoneutral environment, 12-18 hours after eating a meal is called Basal Energy requirement or Basal Metabolic Rate (BMR). Well since it would be very hard for the average person to find themselves in a thermoneutral environment and in the supine position at the same time, being able to accurately calculate your BMR can be quite challenging. The next best method to calculate the total number of calories that you should consume on a daily basis is Resting Metabolic Rate (RMR). RMR is similar to BMR, however the calculation to arrive at your RMR is less complicated. Your RMR is simply your metabolic rate calculated 4 hours after a meal, while you are in a rested state. There is a link to an RMR calculator in the resources section of this book. Knowing your RMR is needed to calculate the number of calories you should consume in a day. Not knowing what your RMR is, can be the difference from having a very successful exercise or weight loss program to a program in which you waste your time, money and effort and get little to no results.

Last but not least is the Total Daily Energy Expenditure or TDEE for short. TDEE is the amount of energy (calories) that is needed for your body to function in a day. Considering that TDEE is made up of three components, TDEE =RMR+Thermic effect of food+Thermic effect of physical activity, your TDEE can fluctuate every day. Your RMR accounts for the largest portion of the TDEE equation at 70%, while the Thermic Effect of Food (Thermic Effect of Food(TEF)-The amount of energy expended above RMR as a result of digesting food for storage and use.) accounts for 10% and the Thermic Effect of Physical Activity (Thermic Effect of Physical Activity-The amount of energy expended above RMR and TEF associated with all forms of physical activity.) accounts for 20%.

Factors that affect your metabolic rate
Genetics
Gender
Age
Weight
Height
Body-fat percentage
Diet nutrition
Body Temperature
External Temperature
Glands or hypothalamus
Exercise

Calculating your TDEE is an essential part of any exercise program. Anyone familiar with certain high intensity Workout Videos are probably familiar with the Harris & Benedict equation which is included in the reading material for these videos. Unfortunately, the Harris & Benedict equation, which was created in 1919 and revised in 1984, is not the most accurate method of calculating how many calories that you should consume on a daily basis. The Harris & Benedict equation only shows accuracy up to 81% of the time in non-obese people. This in itself is a significant problem. Even the slightest miscalculation could result in weight gain instead of weight loss or weight loss instead of weight gain. For example, if your TDEE is calculated to be 2500 calories per day, a 5% miscalculation is equal to a 45,500 calories or a 13 lbs. annual gain or loss.

The most accurate method for calculating your TDEE is by using a formula which includes your bodyfat percentage. The Katch-McArdle and Cunningham formulas use your body fat percentage and the amount of lean mass that you have to determine how many calories you should consume on a daily basis. These formulas are the most accurate method of calculating your TDEE. Why should you use this formula over the other formulas? This is simply because, fat free mass (muscle) accounts for almost 80% of the variation that is seen in resting metabolic rates (RMR) calculated by using formulas like the Harris and Benedict.

There is also evidence which suggests that an increase in lean mass provides significant increases in daily caloric expenditure. In layman's terms, this just means that someone with a higher percentage of lean mass compared to fat mass can metabolize substrates at a higher rate than someone with a higher percentage of fat mass compared to lean mass. There is a Katch-McArdle calculator located in the resources section of this book.

You should also know that calculating how many calories you should consume is not an exact science. There are a number of factors (table to the right) which can affect your metabolic rate and how well your body metabolizes substrates.

Weight loss or Weight gain tip-In order to lose weight you must create an energy (calories) deficit by increasing your physical activity (thermic effect of physical activity) or by reducing your caloric intake. Utilizing a combination of both is the most preferred method. After you calculate your TDEE, you should subtract 300-500 calories from your TDEE for weight loss and for weight gain, you should add 500-800 calories to your TDEE. So remember, to lose 1 lb. of weight you must burn 3,500 calories. If you create a daily deficit of 500 calories, then you'll lose 1 lb. per week!!! ACSM recommends a weight loss of .5-2 lbs. per week as a healthy and realistic expectation.

Metabolic rate is proportional to the amount of lean mass your body has. This means that the more muscle mass that you have, the faster your body metabolizes the carbohydrates, fats and proteins that you consume.

Macronutrients

The term macronutrients are just a scientific term for carbohydrates, proteins and fats. The prefix "macro" means that these nutrients are needed in large amounts. Macronutrients are needed for growth, metabolism and normal body functions.

Carbohydrates

Carbohydrates seem to be one of the most misunderstood of the three macronutrients. With all of the hoopla about low carbohydrate foods, snacks and diets, carbohydrates have gotten a bad name. Carbohydrates are the main source of energy for our body. Did you know that your brain needs a certain amount of glucose (stored carbohydrates) in order to function properly? Because the cells of your brain are always in a state of metabolic activity, your brain cells need two times the energy that other cells in your body need. Now how do you think your brain will perform on a no carbohydrate or low carbohydrate diet? Without sufficient glucose you'll experience mental fatigue which leads to muscle fatigue. When digested, carbohydrates become glucose and glucose is stored in your body as glycogen. Your body can only store so much glycogen, so carbohydrates should be consumed on a frequent basis. Carbohydrates are found in several different forms. These forms have various properties and benefits and can serve different purposes. There are varying opinions regarding the use of the current titles of complex vs simple. Currently there are some professional associations that recommend classifying carbohydrates by their glycemic index. There is more on the glycemic index, later in this chapter. All carbohydrates provide 4 calories of energy for every gram of carbohydrate.

Complex carbohydrates

As mentioned earlier, there are several types of carbohydrates. The most beneficial carbohydrate is called a "complex carbohydrate". Complex carbohydrates are called complex because they contain many molecules of connected sugars and can be full of dietary fiber. Complex carbohydrates are made from three or more monosaccharides and are called polysaccharides and oligosaccharides.

Dietary fiber is a carbohydrate that cannot be digested but is good because it has been known to lower fat and cholesterol absorption, improves sugar control and reduces the risk of colon cancer and heart disease. Men should get 38 grams of fiber per day and women should consume around 25 grams of fiber per day. Fiber helps you to make regular trips to the restroom as well. You'll find that fiber may cause your body to produce more gas than usual. Complex carbohydrates are found in food like beans, peas, whole grains, oatmeal, and potatoes. Complex carbohydrates also contain many vitamins and minerals. When consumed complex carbohydrates are digested slowly and work to even out your energy level throughout the day.

Simple carbohydrates

Simple carbohydrates (sugars) also known as monosaccharides and disaccharides can be found in the form of foods like simple table sugar, maple syrup, soda, candy, jellies and honey. Simple carbohydrates are digested much faster than complex carbohydrates which means that your energy level will spike rapidly and then decline rapidly as well. Simple carbohydrates lack the level of vitamins, minerals and fiber that are found in complex carbohydrates, making the nutritional value of simple carbohydrates low.
However simple sugars aren't all that bad. If you need to quickly "carb up", simple sugars can be the fix. Those with diabetes should take precautionary measures and consult with a doctor.

Inflammation and sugar

It is important to note that sugar has been linked to inflammation. Inflammation is your body's way of fighting infection or a response to injury. Your body sends immune cells and nutrients to the injured or infected area. You may notice inflammation when an injury turns red and starts to swell. The injured area may also feel a bit warm. This is your body's natural and healthy way to fix itself. Inflammation becomes harmful when it doesn't shut down and becomes chronic. Recent research has shown that sugar exaggerates the chronic inflammatory response because it can be an irritant.

Why should I eat every three hours?

I'm sure that you've heard people say that you should eat every three hours. Most people think it is because eating every three hours speeds up your metabolism. Well.... not really. The reason that you should eat every three hours is because blood sugar reaches its peak around 1 hour after eating a meal and then after 2 hours your blood sugar returns to the pre-meal level. Not eating a meal after 3 hours causes your body to go into a deficit and you will start to experience mental and then muscle fatigue.[32] This is because your central nervous system (brain) needs glucose in order to function.[35] Your body's ability to store carbohydrates is limited. When your body does store glucose it stores it in a form called "glycogen".

Glycemic Index/Glycemic Load

As mentioned earlier in this chapter, when there is an increase in insulin secretion, the corresponding action is an increase in the uptake and storage of carbohydrates. Those who are concerned about losing weight and/or managing their glucose levels should pay particular attention to this section. The glycemic index (GI) created in 1980, is an attempt to quantify the blood glucose response to carbohydrates over a two-hour period after ingestion. For those who are focused on weight loss, it is important to know that foods with a high GI can increase the uptake of carbohydrates and storage of fat. The GI ranks foods on a scale from 0 to 100. Foods with a low GI like oatmeal, peas and lentils only slightly raise glucose levels and are digested and absorbed slowly, whereas foods that have a high GI like pineapple, white rice and white bread, increase glucose levels rapidly and are absorbed and digested rapidly. The GI is an estimation. There are other factors that contribute to how carbohydrates may affect your body. The time that carbohydrates are consumed, the type of carbohydrate and the presence of fats and proteins are all factors that may affect how carbohydrates affect your blood glucose.

Because the GI compares carbohydrates on a per gram basis and does not take into account the full impact of the total amount of a meal's carbohydrates has on the body and blood sugar, the Glycemic Load (GL) was created. The GL is the result of multiplying the GI by the amount of carbohydrates in a serving and then dividing this number by 100. Recent research suggests that using the GL as a barometer for dietary guidance can play a significant role in weight loss. Eating foods that have a low GL can reduce fluctuations in glycemic responses and control blood glucose levels which can ultimately result in higher episodes of fat oxidation (fat loss) when compared to high GL meals.

Research has shown that the ingestion of low GI foods prior to exercise cause an increase in free fatty acid oxidation (fat loss) and possibly better maintenance of plasma glucose concentrations, which ultimately leads to a more sustained carbohydrate availability during exercise.

It is important to replenish carbohydrate stores after exercise. It is suggested that a carbohydrate intake of 2 grams carbohydrates/kg of body mass post exercise is sufficient. Increases in fat oxidation were also found after ingesting a single meal post exercise versus snacking on food over a longer duration of time. The rule of thumb is to ingest a high GI meal post exercise in order to increase a glucose response and ingest a low GI meal pre-exercise to burn body fat (fat oxidation).[36]

Even though there is ample evidence to prove that the consumption of low GI meals has shown to help people to lose weight, consuming large quantities of low GI meals can still result in weight gain if the total calories exceed the total amount of calories that a person should consume to maintain their current weight or to lose weight. In other words, the simple principle of more calories in, and less calories burned equals weight gain, still applies.

Muscle building tip-If you are supplementing with creatine, take creatine with a simple, fast digesting sugar based drink made from maltose, glucose or dextrose. This method spikes your insulin levels which can boost creatine absorption levels by 60%.[37]

Drink chocolate milk after your workout...well not so fast...

Yes, we've all seen the marketing campaigns touting chocolate milk as an excellent post workout recovery drink. Some of these campaigns even claim that chocolate milk beats out Gatorade as a post exercise recovery drink. This particular claim certainly got people's attention. Joel Stanger, an Exercise Physiologist at Indiana University and competitive swimmer, starting giving his 20-something aged swimmers chocolate milk as a post recovery drink.[38] He found the levels of stored glycogen had increased after drinking chocolate milk as compared to other carbohydrate drinks like Gatorade.

Here's what they aren't telling you. Each cup of chocolate milk contains 50% carbohydrates, 35% fats and 15% protein. Chocolate milk has a moderate glycemic index number of 49, but has a high glycemic load number of 88. As stated earlier in this chapter, foods that have a high GI and/or GL will increase the storage of carbohydrates and fats. If you are in a weight loss program, drinking chocolate milk after a workout might not be the best choice.

Protein

Remember when you would hear about people drinking raw eggs so that they could get the highest concentration of protein in their bodies? If you watched any media about the Floyd Mayweather vs. Juan Manuel Marquez fight in 2009, Juan actually takes it a step further and uses a home remedy in an attempt to increase the amount of protein in his body. You'll have to use Google to get the details on that. Both of these examples are extreme and largely refuted methods of ways to increase protein levels within the body. These methods certainly don't produce any better results than eating a 6 oz. piece of grilled chicken. On average, protein by far is one of the least consumed, but highly important of the three macronutrients.

By in large, the average diet is filled with foods consisting of mostly carbohydrates and fats and almost void of any protein. The lack of consuming the appropriate amount of protein can eventually lead to several health issues to include osteoporosis, advanced sarcopenia, muscle cramping or edema (swelling). Unlike carbohydrates and fats, protein is not a primary source of energy, even though proteins contain 4 calories per gram, just like carbohydrates. So why is protein important? Most importantly, protein is necessary for tissue growth and maintenance. Proteins are important for hormone production, enzyme and protein synthesis. Proteins can also help to control the fluid balance between the blood and surrounding tissues, which helps you to maintain blood volume and sweat rates during exercise. Now before you go run out to GNC or Vitamin Shoppe to buy a tub of protein, it's important to understand the various aspects of protein.

Protein quality

Protein quality is determined by the presence of essential and nonessential proteins. Essential proteins are proteins that are "essential" however our bodies are unable to produce them. This means that we have to eat these proteins in order to make them present in our bodies. Non-essential proteins are proteins that our bodies can make.[39] Not to confuse you any longer, but a complete protein contains all of the essential proteins and an incomplete protein doesn't. Complete proteins are found in animal based food products or proteins. Foods such as fish, steak, milk, eggs, whey, and casein contain all the essential proteins. Incomplete proteins are found in plant based food products or proteins, with the exception of soy. There is an ongoing debate on whether protein from hemp and quinoa are complete or incomplete, but both can be an added bonus to anyone's nutritional plan. Those who are vegetarian are at a higher risk of inadequate protein intake as compared to their meat eating counterparts.

Essential Proteins		
Histidine	Isoleucine	Leucine
Valine	Lysine	Methionine
Phenylalanyl	Threonine	Tryptophan
Non-Essential Proteins		
Alanine	Arginine	Asparagine
Aspartic Acid	Cysteine	Glutamic Acid
Glutamine	Glycine	Proline
Serine	Tyrosine	

However, with proper planning, vegetarians can create a nutrition plan that gives them the essential proteins that are necessary for proper body function.

So the next question that you may be asking is, "How much protein should I be consuming?"

There is also an ongoing debate about how much protein a person should consume. Protein intake can vary by age, gender and/or activity level. The American College of Sports Medicine (ACSM) states that the average person should consume .8 grams of protein per kilogram of body weight. ACSM also states that endurance athletes should consume 1.6 -1.7 grams of protein per kilogram of body weight or no more than 10-15% of total energy expenditure.[40]

So let's take a look at two different methods to calculate your total daily protein consumption. Using ACSM's guidance, a 200 lbs. person who has an average activity level should consume 73 grams (200/2.2=90.9 and 90.9 x .8) or 291 calories of protein per day. Protein consumption levels can also be determined by using the Katch McArdle method for calculating TDEE. Since the Katch McArdle method uses your body fat percentage to calculate the total amount of calories to consume, it is the most accurate. Using the Katch McArdle method, a 200 lbs. person with 20% body fat who is moderately active should consume 2,106 calories per day which equates to 210.6 calories (53 grams) to 315.9 calories (79 grams) or 10-15% of TDEE. However, in 2013, ACSM updated its guideline on protein intake to 10-35% of TDEE. Using ACSM's updated guideline, in this example protein intake reaches 737 calories (184 grams) at 35% of TDEE.

So now, let's discuss protein supplementation. Many people opt to supplement their protein consumption by using a protein powder. It is important to know the facts about protein powders so that you can decide which protein works best for your situation.

Protein subtypes

There are four main protein subtypes; concentrate, Isolate, hydrolyzed and micellar.[41] These subtypes vary based on quality, absorption rate and price.

Concentrate

Concentrate protein by comparison, is the lowest quality of protein that you can buy. Concentrate protein is processed more than other subtypes of protein and yields the lowest percent of protein at 70%-80%. Concentrate protein is not particularly void of any redeeming qualities, it's just not the best quality of protein. Concentrate protein is the lowest costing of the four sub-type, so you'll normally find this type of protein in very large containers. Concentrate protein tends to have more "stuff" mixed in with it, like carbohydrates and fats. Speaking from my own personal experience, I consistently used concentrate protein, well before I knew about and understood other protein subtypes. I believe that I was still able to achieve my fitness and athletic performance goals while supplementing with concentrate proteins.

Isolate

Moving up the ladder is isolate protein. Isolate protein yields 90%-94% protein, but is more expensive to buy than concentrate. If you choose an isolate, make sure that you read the label. You'll find that some isolates are mixed with concentrate and the label doesn't tell you how much of the protein powder is concentrate or how much is isolate. You could be buying mostly concentrate, but because there is some isolate mixed in with it, the manufacturer could put isolate on the label and charge you a similar price that you might pay for 100% isolate.

Hydrolysate or Hydrolyzed

Now it's time to crack open the wallet! Hydrolyzed protein is the most expensive protein that you can buy. However, hydrolyzed almost requires no further breakdown of the protein by your body's enzymes and enters your bloodstream faster than concentrate and isolate. Again, before you buy, make sure you read the ingredients and make sure the label states 100% hydrolyzed.

Micellar

Because of the way it is processed, micellar is readily digested and absorbed into the bloodstream. This protein is not altered or damaged by physical and chemical processes that cause damage to the protein's structure. Micellar protein typically cost more than other protein subtypes.

Biological Value of protein

Before we start down the path of breaking down the various types of protein supplements, it's important to know and understand a term called the "biological value" of protein. The biological value (BV) is a measure of the proportion of absorbed protein from a food which becomes incorporated into the proteins of the organism's body.[42] In layman's terms, BV is the measure of how well the body can absorb and utilize a protein. This measure quantifies how readily the digested protein can be used in protein synthesis in the cells of the organism. The higher the BV the better the protein. There are other methods that measure the effectiveness or usability of protein, but the BV value is the most common. For example, a whole egg has a BV of 100, which is on the upper end of the range. White flour has a BV of 41.

Whey protein

Whey protein is an animal based protein and has the highest concentration of the 9 essential amino acids. Whey to go!!!! I know...I couldn't resist. :) Out of all the proteins, Whey protein is digested the fastest. You can purchase Whey in a concentrate, isolate or hydrolyzed form. Believe it or not, Whey protein has a BV of 104 to 159 depending on whether the Whey protein is concentrate or isolate. Whey works best either before a workout or shortly after a workout. However, to increase your overall protein consumption, consuming whey protein during the day is recommended as well.

Soy protein

Soy protein is a plant based protein, however unlike other plant based proteins, it contains all of the 9 essential amino acids. Soy isolate has a BV of 74, much lower than whey. However, soy has a higher concentration of
arginine and glutamine than whey or casein protein. Soy can be used for muscle recovery and for consumption throughout the day.

Casein protein

One of the most neglected and unheard of proteins is casein. Casein performs like no other and should certainly get a second look. Casein is an animal based product and it makes up 80% of the protein content of cow's milk. Casein has a BV of 77, however it performs in a much different way than it's animal and plant based protein counterparts. Casein is insoluble and actually forms small globules or "gel" which takes longer to digest. Understanding that your body is always in two states, Anabolic (building) or catabolic (breaking down), casein actually slows down the catabolic state and the resulting breakdown of muscle tissue.

Therefore, casein is great for consumption right before bed. In a 2011 study, casein proved to have a good effect on the satiety level of the research subjects.[11] The study found that casein lowered the amount of food consumption in test subjects because it made them feel full.

Hemp protein

Hemp protein is mostly used by vegetarians, but is gaining popularity with steadfast meat eaters. Hemp however does not have the same protein content as its animal based protein comparators. Hemp protein has a BV of around 50. The great thing about hemp protein is that is has more fiber than other proteins. On average hemp can cost $20 for 16 ounces of product. This makes hemp somewhat pricier than the most popular animal based or plant based proteins like whey and soy.

When should I consume protein?

Protein should always be a normal part of each meal that is consumed throughout the day. According to ACSM, protein turnover is increased with resistance training for up to 48 hours in people beginning a new resistance training program.[40] ACSM also quotes several studies which have demonstrated that protein ingestion after a bout of resistance training stimulates muscle protein synthesis for up to three hours. Studies also show that failing to consume protein after exercise may limit protein synthesis and therefore limit potential progress in lean muscle tissue development. Research also suggests that consuming protein one (1) hour after exercise has the greatest influence on resistance training adaptations. This period immediately after exercise is commonly called the "anabolic window" or "metabolic window". It is thought that ingesting protein and carbohydrates within this "window" can aid in the increase in building muscle mass.

From my own training experience, I've found that ingesting a specific ratio of carbohydrates, fats, and proteins within 30-45 minutes of my workouts, has aided in building muscle mass and increasing performance for the future days ahead. Since whey protein is a fast absorbing protein, I'll normally consume a higher proportion of whey than any other type of protein, within this window of time.

Fats

This a topic that also seems to confuse the average consumer or health enthusiast. I often hear people say, "But it's good fat!". There is an ongoing debate in the health and fitness community on whether the so called "bad" fat is actually bad. However, you slice it, the calories from the good fat or the bad fat is the same. As compared to proteins and carbohydrates, fats contain 9 calories for each gram, more than double its macronutrient counterparts. Knowing this information will be very important as we move to the section that describes how to read food labels. Fats or lipids, as it is commonly called, certainly have some good qualities though. Stored body fat protects organs against sudden concussive forces and provides insulation. Fat in food gives our food flavor and carries essential vitamins such as A, D, E, and K. Lipids include triglycerides, phospholipids and cholesterol. If a lipid is solid at room temperature, then it is fat. If a lipid is a liquid at room temperature, then it is an oil.

When we eat too many calories our body stores the excess fat (calories) in adipose tissue for release into the bloodstream as free fatty acids. A heavy accumulation of body fat in adipose tissue is highly correlated with atherosclerosis, a process in which the arterial wall becomes thickened leading to a narrowing of the lumen in the artery. This can cause coronary heart disease, a stroke or a myocardial infarction (heart attack). There are other issues that can lead to this problem to include an elevated serum cholesterol and triglycerides, high blood pressure and cigarette smoke.

I'm sure that when you've gone to the doctor and gotten bloodwork (lipid panel) completed, that the terms TC, HDL, and LDL were discussed or printed on the paperwork that you received. Total Serum cholesterol (TC) is the sum of all forms of cholesterol in the blood and is broken up into "good" lipids called high density lipoproteins (HDL) and "bad" lipids called low density lipoproteins (LDL). An HDL level greater than 60mg/dL is considered good and offers protection against heart disease. The concentration of HDL can be influenced by heredity, gender, exercise and diet. Dyslipidemia is an abnormal amount of lipids in the blood, however most people are affected by a high level of lipids in the blood called hyperlipidemia. An LDL level of equal to or greater than 130 mg/dL or a total serum cholesterol level of greater than or equal to 200 mg/dl is a risk factor for cardiovascular disease. Polyunsaturated fat (vegetable/cereal/corn oil) and monounsaturated fat (olive/canola oil) tend to lower blood cholesterol, while saturated fatty acids (meat/dairy) tend to increase serum cholesterol. Fats from animals have a higher proportion of saturated fat and fat from plants have a higher proportion of monounsaturated and/or polyunsaturated fat (coconut, palm kernel and palm oil excluded).

A few years ago ACSM recommended a fat intake of no more than 35% of the total calories that adults consume. However, ACSM updated its recommendation in 2013, after realizing that the epidemic of obesity continues to climb. ACSM lowered its recommendation from 35% to 25% or less, including recommending a diet consisting of less than 10% saturated fat.

Saturated fat

I've recently read several cookbooks, including paleo diet books, which suggest that as long as you consume organic unrefined forms of saturated fat in any amount, you're eating healthy. Well this is partly true. The problem with saturated fat is that we tend to consume too much of it. Saturated fat is basically fat that consists of triglycerides and is saturated with "hydrogen". High levels of triglycerides in the bloodstream have been linked to heart disease and stroke. Research has shown that saturated fats contribute to hardening of the arteries by increasing cholesterol levels. Saturated fat is also linked to an increase in total cholesterol and LDL cholesterol which are risk factors for cardiovascular disease. Since our body makes enough saturated fat to meet our physiological needs, there is no dietary requirement for saturated fat. This means that if you can get away with eating a diet void of saturated fats, then you are much better off. [12] Some foods that are major sources of saturated fat are cheese, pizza, grain based desserts, dairy based desserts, sausage, franks, bacon and ribs. The American Heart Association recommends that no more than 7% of your daily caloric intake should consist of saturated fats.

Unsaturated fat

Unsaturated fats are monounsaturated fat, polyunsaturated fat and trans fat. Chemically speaking monounsaturated is a fatty acid chain that contains one double bond and polyunsaturated fat contains more than one double bond. Where double bonds are formed hydrogen atoms are eliminated, hence the name "unsaturated".

Monounsaturated fat

Monounsaturated fats can help to reduce bad cholesterol levels and can also provide nutrients to help develop and maintain your body's cells.[43] Monounsaturated fats can be found in olive oil, canola oil, peanut oil and sesame oil.

Polyunsaturated fat

Polyunsaturated fat (fatty acids) have two or more double bonds. The good thing about polyunsaturated fat is that it provides essential fats like omega-6 and omega-3, fats that your body can't produce itself. Polyunsaturated fats can help to reduce cholesterol levels thereby reducing your risk for cardiovascular disease and stroke.[44] Foods that are high in polyunsaturated fat include soybean oil, corn oil, sunflower oil, salmon, mackerel, herring and trout.[13] Although polyunsaturated fat has some great qualities, remember that all fats have 9 calories for every gram of fat. So don't overdo it!

Trans fat

According to the Mayo Clinic, Trans fat is considered by many doctors to be the worst type of fat you can eat.[45] Trans-fat raises your LDL(bad) cholesterol and lowers your HDL (good) cholesterol.[14] Trans-fat is formed naturally by cows and other grazing animals. As a result of an industrial process, hydrogen is added to vegetable oil, which causes the oil to become solid at room temperature. This partially hydrogenated oil increases the shelf life of the foods that it is made from. Foods that have been deep fried probably have been cooked in hydrogenated vegetable oil. Trans fat can be found in cakes, cookies, pie crusts, french fries, corn/tortilla chips, non-dairy coffee creamer, frozen pizza, canned biscuits and microwave popcorn. Wow, is there anything else that we could possibly eat? Food manufacturers and producers in the United States are allowed to label their products as having 0 trans-fat, even if the food contains .5 grams of trans fat in a serving. However, in 2015, the Food and Drug Administration announced that companies that use trans-fat have 3 years to phase out the once thought of "super fat". If you read a food label and the words hydrogenated or partially hydrogenated appear, then the food contains trans fats. You should attempt to eat a healthy diet that is free of trans fats.

How to read a food label

I think that it is safe to say that most people, at least in the United States, purchase the majority of their food from a grocery store or commissary. Even though we spend a considerable amount of time in these establishments, it still amazes me how much we don't know about the food that we purchase from these places and how these foods can affect our health.

During one of my frequent excursions, I was on a flight returning to Atlanta from New York, when I met two ladies from South Georgia. As I whipped out my books to read, I felt a tap on my shoulder. One of these ladies apparently saw some of the book titles that I was about to read. She shyly asks, "Are you an athlete or trainer?". Little did I know that this inquiry would result in a conversation that would last almost the entire flight duration, from the wheels up in New York to the wheels down in Atlanta. Not to bore you with all the details of our conversation, but the topic that took the most time to discuss revolved around nutrition. I asked one of the ladies to show me some food that she had purchased from the store in the airport, that she thought was healthy. She pulled out a Nature Valley bar that was labeled as a Protein Chewy Bar. Now before I get some sort of nasty gram from Nature Valley, let me say that I can eat these bars like there is no tomorrow. However, I want to point out to my readers, that labels can be deceiving. If you recall from our previous discussion on macronutrients and the ACSM recommended daily intake percentages, carbohydrates contain 4 calories per gram, protein contains 4 calories per gram and fats contain 9 calories per gram. ACSM also recommends a macronutrient breakdown of 10-35% protein, less than 30% fat and 45-65% carbohydrates. So let's do the math! According to Nature Valley's food label, 1 bar contains 190 calories which is derived from 108 calories of fat (12 grams x9 calories), 40 calories of protein (10 grams x4 calories) and 36 calories of carbohydrates (9 grams x 4 calories). If food contains 5 grams of fiber or more, then you can subtract 5 grams or more from the total amount of carbohydrates. You can also see that saturated fat makes up almost 30% of the total fat of this product (3.5grams/12 grams=29.2%). And we already know about saturated fat.

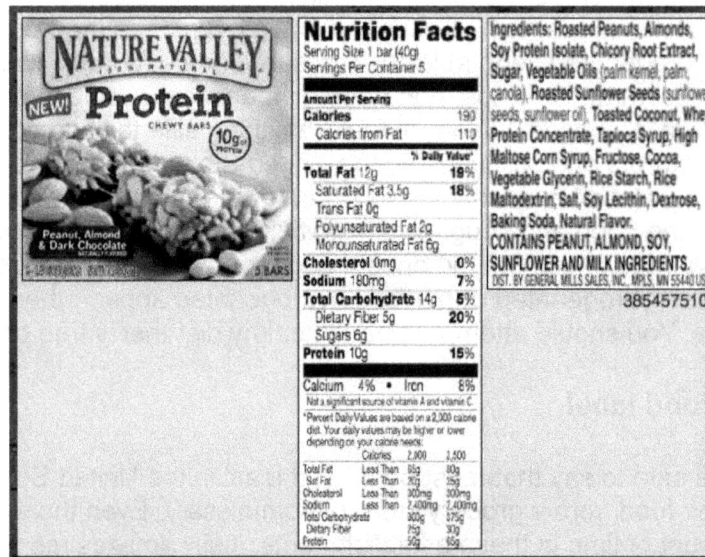

So now let's take a look at the macronutrient breakdown of the Nature Valley Chewy Bar. As the chart to the right shows, fats make up almost 60% of the total calories in this product. Just remember, the box and the individual product are labeled "Protein". Now, take a look at the comparison chart on the lower right. You can compare the macronutrient percentage breakdown to the ACSM recommendations and my diet.

Macronutrient Breakdown Nature Valley Chewy Bar		
	# of calories	% of total calories
Fats	108	59%
Carbohydrates	36	20%
Protein	40	22%
Total	184	

Chewy Bar Macronutrient comparison

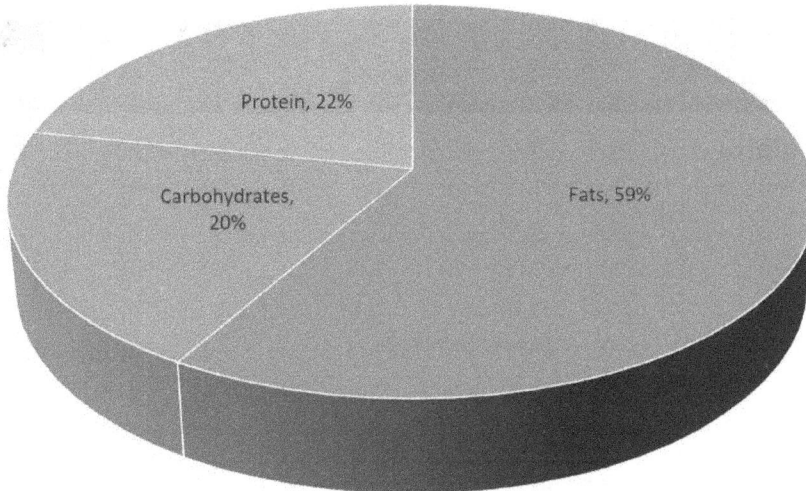

Protein, 22%

Carbohydrates, 20%

Fats, 59%

If you find yourself in a situation where you think you've eaten more than your fair share of fats for the day, you can balance out your daily diet, by lowering your consumption of any additional fatty foods and/0r increase your protein or carbohydrate consumption throughout the day. You can use this method to balance out your macronutrient consumption needs and tailor your diet specifically for you.

Since I don't want to be perceived as picking on Nature Valley, I thought that I would throw in a southern favorite, Chick-Fil-A. Below is the actual nutrition information pulled directly from the Chick-Fil-A website.

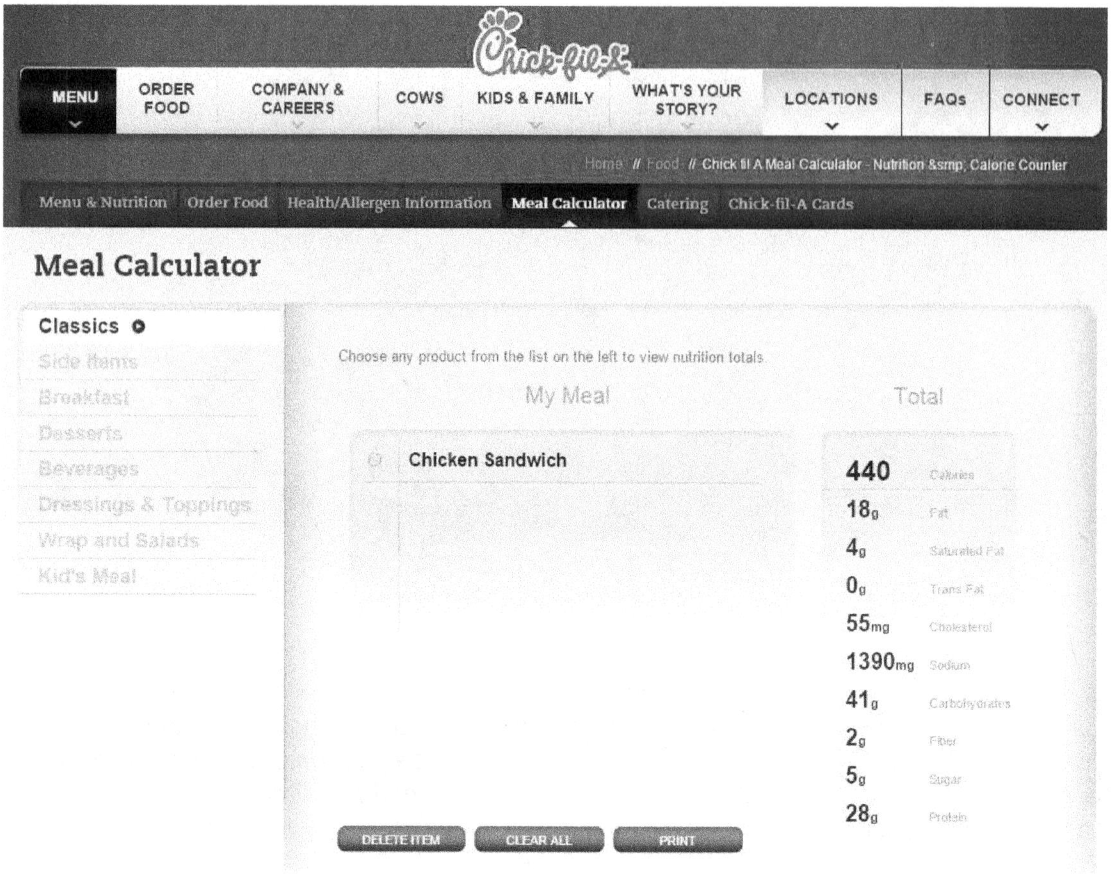

Meal Calculator

Classics ○

Side Items

Breakfast

Desserts

Beverages

Dressings & Toppings

Wrap and Salads

Kid's Meal

Choose any product from the list on the left to view nutrition totals.

My Meal   Total

Chicken Sandwich

440 Calories

18g Fat

4g Saturated Fat

0g Trans Fat

55mg Cholesterol

1390mg Sodium

41g Carbohydrates

2g Fiber

5g Sugar

28g Protein

DELETE ITEM   CLEAR ALL   PRINT

So let's break down the macronutrients of one Chick-fil-A sandwich like we did the Nature Valley bar. According to their website, one Chick-fil-A sandwich contains 162 calories of fat (18 grams x 9 calories), 164 calories of carbohydrates (41 grams x 4 calories) and 112 calories of protein (28 grams x 4 calories). As you can see by the chart below, this sandwich is over 70% carbohydrates and fat. Two important notes to make is that the sodium level in one Chick-fil-A sandwich is almost as high as the recommended daily intake. The National, Heart, Lung and Blood Institutes recommend a daily sodium intake of 1,500 to 2,300 mg/day. As you can see, one Chick-Fil-A sandwich has 1390 mg of sodium. So it's especially important for those who are concerned about health issues like high blood pressure to be able to understand the sodium content of the food that is consumed. The problem is...as we know, who only eats one Chick-fil-A sandwich? I know I didn't. The chart and graph below detail the macronutrient breakdown of one (1) Chick-fil-A sandwich.

Macronutrient	ACSM recommendation	George's Diet	Chick-fil-A label Breakdown
Fats	<30%	20%	37%(162 calories)
Carbohydrates	45-65%	45%	37%(164 calories)
Protein	10-35%	35%	26%(112 calories)

Chick-fil-A sandwich macronutrient breakdown

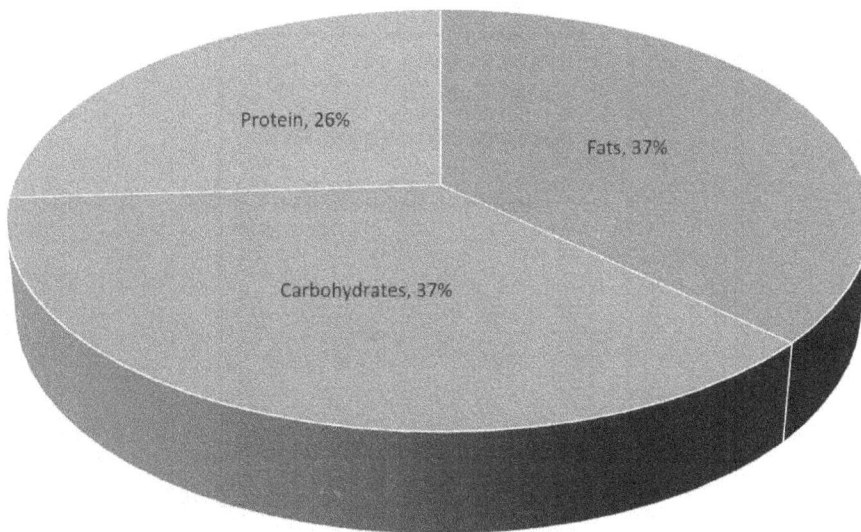

Protein, 26%

Fats, 37%

Carbohydrates, 37%

Misleading food label information

As shown on food labels, a "% Daily Value" is provided for each macronutrient that is listed on the label. In the example to the right 9% is given to the total fat content and 13% is given to the total carbohydrates of this product. Unfortunately, 9% and 13% are not the true values for these two nutrients. The % Daily Value is based on a 2,000 calorie per day diet.[46] The true calorie value of these two nutrients are 22% (fat-54 calories/250 calories) and 65% (carbohydrates-160 calories/250 calories). This is confusing to most people, so it is important to understand that the values that are written on the label are not the true caloric value of each of the macronutrients listed on a label.

Nutrition Facts	
Serving Size ¼ cup (55g)	
Servings Per Container 5	
Amount Per Serving	
Calories 250	Calories from Fat 50
	% Daily Value*
Total Fat 6g	9%
Saturated Fat 0.5g	3%
Cholesterol <5mg	<2%
Sodium 200mg	8%
Total Carbohydrate 40g	13%
Dietary Fiber 4g	16%
Sugars 18g	
Protein 9g	18%
Vitamin A 25% • Vitamin C 50% • Calcium 30% • Iron 25%	
*Percent Daily Values based on a 2,000 Calorie diet.	

Portion control

Portion distortion is defined as "an upward shift in the size and calorie count of a serving of a particular food served to the general public, especially in the fast food industry". Over the last 40 years the food portion sizes found in restaurants and fast food chains have continued to increase in size. Some claim that because of the increase in food portions the incidence of obesity has raised to a worldwide epidemic. Even the size of plates has increased over the same time period. In the 1960's a regular plate was 9 inches in diameter. 20 years later an inch was added making a regular plate 10 inches in diameter. Fast forward another 20+ years and the average plate is found to be between 11 and 12 inches in diameter. [47]

If you watched the movie Supersize me, you saw the main character, Morgan Spurlock, gorge himself on Big Macs, Double cheeseburgers, large fries and every other food item that was on the McDonald's menu. As a result of his 30-day experiment, he gained 30 lbs. and his cholesterol level went from 165 mg/dL to 225 mg/dL during this period. [48]
In 2013, Mayor Michael Bloomberg attempted to make the sale of sodas over 16 ounces in the state of New York, illegal. The legal attempt was eventually thwarted when the state's highest court found that the Mayor and the Department of Health and Mental Hygiene had overstepped their legal authority. [49]

Although I don't agree with these extreme examples of bringing awareness to certain food products that have the potential to increase our waistlines and potentially can be harmful to our health, the message that both of these efforts sends certainly hold some truth. Plainly put. We eat too much and move too little. As compared to many other countries, the United States makes low cost, high calorie, low nutrient foods easily accessible in almost every corner of the country. For some neighborhoods this is the only type of food that is readily accessible or within a local commuting distance.

Portion control allows a person to manage the amount of food that is consumed at every meal. As discussed throughout this chapter, there are several different methods that have helped people to achieve success in their attempts to reign in their waistlines.

Your plate

The first method is the easiest and cheapest way to manage food consumption. Take a regular sized plate (10") and visually draw two lines, dividing the plate in half and then dividing the lower half by 30% and 20%. 50% of your plate should be filled with vegetables like corn, broccoli, or green beans. 30% of your plate should be reserved for proteins like chicken or fish. 20% of your plate should be filled with carbohydrates (complex) like brown rice, quinoa, or freekah. The height of the food on your plate should not exceed ½ inch to 1 inch. You can use this method to control food portion sizes for each meal that you consume throughout the day. Please remember, liquids such as sodas, sweetened tea or other sugary drinks, adds to the number of calories that are consumed each day.

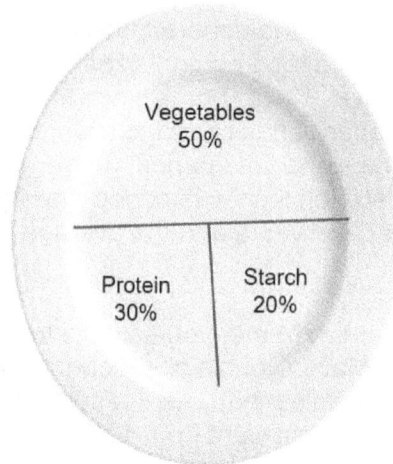

Measured containers

Another method that has shown some success in helping people to control the amount of food that is consumed, is to use portion control containers. Several companies offer specific sized plastic containers to store certain types of food, which help you to determine the right amount of food to consume. These containers are relatively inexpensive with prices ranging from $10 to $30 per set. Sets can be ordered online or at your nearest health food store or grocery store.

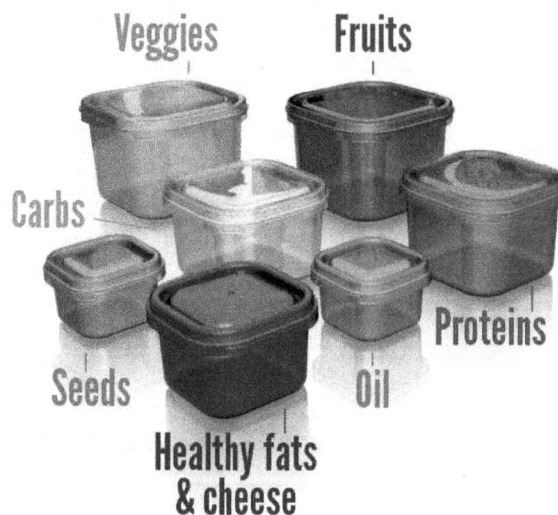

Your hand

The third and most cost effective method is to simply use your hand as a measuring device. Each of the food groups can be represented by a part of your hand. For example, your palm is about the size of a 3-4-ounce piece of chicken or fish. Your thumb is almost the size of 1-2 tablespoons; just the right size for a taste of peanut butter, sour cream or salad dressing. One cup is approximately the size of your fist; making this the right size for fruit or ice cream.

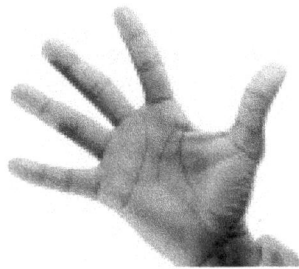

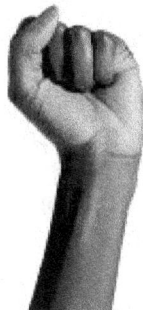

Eating healthy foods in.....is much cheaper than eating non-healthy foods out.

Unfortunately, there is a common misperception that it costs more to eat healthy, than it is to eat unhealthy. If you take a stroll down the seafood aisle of Whole Foods, which normally boasts $20-$25/lb. for salmon, I can certainly understand why many people think this way. However, this perception couldn't be farther from the truth.

The United States Department of Agriculture (USDA) publishes a monthly document titled, "Official USDA Food Plans: Cost of Food at Home at Four Levels"50. These monthly line item documents show the weekly and monthly cost of food plans for eating in, based on age and gender. For a moderate plan, it cost $205.60 per week or $29.37 per day, to feed a family of four. In contrast, according to data provided by Visa, on average, men spend $21 and women spend $14 on lunch outside the home.[51] Multiply these numbers by the number of times a person may eat out and then multiply that number by the number of total family members, and the annual bill can skyrocket. The data from Visa's survey, also showed that those who make less than $50,000 annually spend $11.70 on lunch outside the home and those who make over $50,000 only spend $9.60.

As you can see, eating out certainly doesn't save you any money when compared to the cost of food prepared in the home. Generally speaking, food prepared in the home can also be a much healthier option than eating fast food. If prepared well, food cooked in the home can be a low fat, high nutrient dense option. Another benefit of preparing meals at home is having the ability to spend more quality time with your family. Have you ever tried to cook a meal with a family member? It's quite the experience and can certainly bring you closer together, especially if you have a small kitchen.

Organic foods vs. conventional foods.

If you don't mind sacrificing a little taste for value, conventionally made foods like meat, milk, peas, salmon, tuna and chicken can be a cheaper, but still nutritious option to buying organic foods. There are several studies from the CDC, USDA, American Cancer Society, WebMD and other credible organizations that don't support the notion that organic foods are much better for you than conventional foods. Where there might be some added benefit that organic foods might offer over conventional foods, the net effect is negligible. Based on my own experience with developing nutrition plans for athletic performance and competition preparation, I'd have to agree with the findings of these organizations. Considering that most of my clients and the people who I come into contact with, can't afford to eat organic foods on a daily basis, conventional foods have shown to be a healthy option. You can read more about organic foods vs conventional goods by going to the resources page of this book.

Average cost

$1-$3/meal cooked in the home

VS.

$7-$10/fast food meal

So where do I shop to get healthy low cost food?

Believe it or not, I get the most out of my money by shopping at Costco, Sam's Club and Walmart. I can purchase large amounts of common items like fish, chicken, vegetables, and almond milk, much cheaper, at these well-known discount locations than I can at the normal grocery chains that are in my neighborhood. Even if you have to travel a few miles past your local grocery store to reach one of these places, the savings that you will experience makes the trip well worth it.

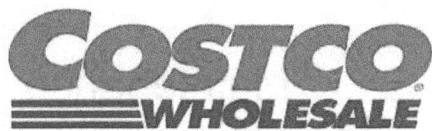

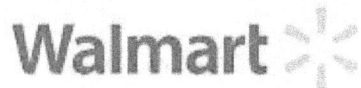

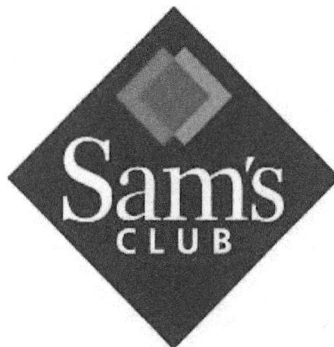

Chapter 4

Maintenance
(Developing your own fitness programs.)

Good things come to those who.....WORK! Earn it.

George Dorsey

Over my 20 years of being in the health and fitness industry, I've come to realize that people who pursue their health and fitness goals can be placed into five main groups; 1) Newbies, 2) Old school gym heads, 3) Group instruction groupies, 4) Fitness Fad followers, and 5) Guilt driven gym goers.

Even though these groups cover a wide range of demographics, interests, motivations and goals, they all have one thing in common. They all tend to piecemeal their workouts together from things they've read in magazines, television ads, and social media. Others focus their workout efforts from what they may have heard from friends, family and passer byers. Goals are not achieved, gains are not maximized and year after year, specific results are never realized.

When I was a member of a gym in Colorado, I met a middle aged woman named Kelly. Unfortunately, I have to use her real first name, for the simple fact that the name that was given to her by other gym members fits neatly after the noun that precedes it. Her gym name was "Cardio Kelly". Kelly had been a long term member of this gym and she was well known and well liked. When I met Kelly she had just started to switch up her workout routine based on a workout program that she had read about in a magazine. This workout plan focused more on cardiorespiratory (aerobic) exercises and claimed to produce amazing weight loss results. So you may ask why was she given the name of Cardio Kelly? Because of her new found workout plan, Kelly spent no less than 3-4 hours a day, executing a long a tenuous aerobic routine. As time went on, I watched Kelly shrink from a 140 lbs. female to less than 100 lb. frame of skin and bone. Kelly began to lack muscle tone and her face started to look emaciated and pale. Unbeknownst to Kelly her body was in a continuous state of catabolism. In an attempt to maintain some sort of energy balance her body was essentially eating its own tissue to include muscle tissue and any evidence of essential body fat. Kelly started to complain of kidney pain and was later diagnosed with Rhabdomyolysis. Rhabdomyolysis is the breakdown of muscle tissue that leads to muscle fiber contents into the blood. Luckily for Kelly she was able to get the help that she needed which included nutritional guidance, development of an effective and tailored exercise plan and support from other gym members.

Now, Kelly is an extreme example of a person who didn't quite understand the basics of nutrition and health and how physical activity can actually be harmful instead of helpful.
Kelly is an extreme case, but unfortunately she represents the norm. As of April 2015, it is estimated that there are at least 58 million people who hold gym memberships.[52] This number obviously doesn't include those who exercise outdoors or at home. Out of these tens of millions of people, how many do you think are actually qualified and knowledgeable enough to put together a thorough and tailored exercise plan that helps to prevent injury, increase cardiorespiratory capacity, increases/maintains muscle mass,

reduces excess body fat, increases flexibility or range of motion and reduces risk for certain diseases?

The information in this chapter will help give you a basic understanding of how to; assess your overall health and to develop and execute a safe and results oriented exercise plan, based on the principles established by the American College of Sports Medicine, the National Academy of Sports Medicine, from my own experience and education and various other reputable sources. So let's get started.

Before you exercise, get a medical evaluation.

Before you lift one weight and before you take one step on a treadmill, you should make time to get a medical evaluation. According to the American College of Sports Medicine the risk of sudden death caused by a heart attack is higher in adults than in younger individuals. The incidence of heart attack is even higher for sedentary adults who are unaccustomed to frequent exercise. Those who have symptoms of or have been diagnosed with cardiovascular, pulmonary or metabolic disease are at a high risk for a heart attack. Men over the age of 45 and women over the age of 55, those who smoke or who have quit smoking within the last 6 months and those with elevated cholesterol and glucose levels are at a high risk for cardiovascular disease (CVD). If you remember who Jim Fixx and Edmund Burke were and how they died, then you'll know that this is serious topic. Research has shown that the risk for sudden death during vigorous physical activity is estimated at 1 per year for every 15,000 to 18,000 people.[53] [54] Another study raised the estimation to 2.7 events per 10,000 people for men and 6 events for women. Getting a medical evaluation before you start an exercise program, will help you to identify risk factors which could potentially harm you.

For example, Clarence is 54 years old and weighs 168 pounds. Clarence recently went to his primary care physician and found out that he had a resting heart rate of 64 bpm, total serum cholesterol of 187 mg/dL, HDL of 52 mg/dL and a Body Mass Index of 22.8. Clarence is a runner who runs four to seven days per week and has actually completed two marathons within the last year. Clarence's father, died at the age of 77 of a heart attack and his mother died at the age of 81 of cancer. Clarence's physician has never prescribed him any medication. Clarence was found to be at low risk for cardiovascular disease (CVD). Because Clarence is low risk, he can safely participate in physical activity without the supervision of any medical personnel.

Meet Marilyn. Marilyn is 35 years old and a non-smoker. Marilyn recently completed a lipid panel at a free clinic and found out that her total cholesterol was 174 mg/dL. At age 7, Marilyn was diagnosed with Type 1 diabetes and has to take regular insulin injections. Marilyn stays pretty active by teaching a group cardio class three times every week and walks for 45 minutes at least four times per week. Both of Marilyn's parents are in good health. Marilyn is classified as having a high risk for CVD because of her earlier diagnosis of Type 1 diabetes. Because Marilyn is a high risk, Marilyn was supervised by her physician during her exercise sessions, until her physician and her trainer could establish a safe exercise program for her.

So before you pop in that next installment of your favorite high intensity workout video or hop on the elliptical machine you should complete a basic medical evaluation to determine your current and future risk for heart attack, stroke or other physical ailments. A medical evaluation will tell you the types of physical activity that you are allowed to participate in and if any medical supervision is needed. A basic medical evaluation typically starts with a questionnaire and some blood work. A health history questionnaire is designed to highlight if you are at low, medium or high risk for cardiovascular disease or any other medical issues that may potentially cause you harm. A sample health history questionnaire is included in the resources section of this book.

You can use this questionnaire to help determine your risk for CVD or other health issues, prior to starting your exercise regimen. A medical evaluation should also consist of completion of a metabolic and lipid panel. A metabolic panel is a blood test that measures your glucose level, electrolyte, fluid balance, and kidney and liver functions. A lipid panel is a blood test that measures your cholesterol and triglycerides. The chart below displays biomarkers for normal, borderline and high risk. You can use this chart to compare the results of your blood work. However, your physician should be able to go over your results with you when they become available.

	Normal	Borderline High risk	High risk
Total Cholesterol	<200	200-239	$\geq$ 240
LDL Cholesterol	<100	130-159	160-189
HDL Cholesterol*	<40		
Triglycerides	<150	150-199	200-499
Blood pressure Systolic	<120	120-139	140- $\geq$160
Blood pressure Diastolic	<80	80-89	90- $\geq$100
Impaired Fasting glucose*	60-99 mg. dL	100-125	$\geq$125
Impaired glucose tolerance test*	>140 mg/dL-1		>200 mg/dL-1

*>60 mg/dl is a positive factor.

Don't have a primary care physician? That is okay. You can still get a free to low cost evaluation at places like CVS and Walgreens. These companies offer clinic like services to the general public, typically at a reduced cost. You can contact either one of these companies and ask for a metabolic and/or lipid panel. A metabolic panel and lipid panel at Walgreens or CVS can run from $5 to $70 for those without insurance and even less for those with insurance. Walmart tests are considerably cheaper showing recent cost of less than $10 for each panel.

minute
clinic

healthcare
clinic
at select Walgreens

The Clinic
at Walmart

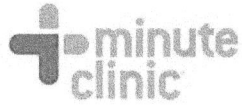

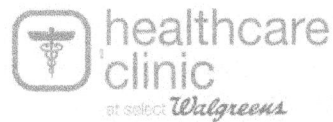

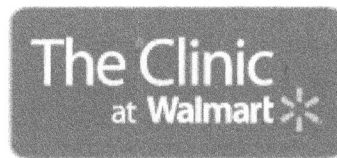

When it comes to getting your blood work completed, there is a new company called Theranos, that deserves a second look. Theranos claims to have reduced the cost of blood testing and also claims to have made the process more efficient. According to their website, all you need to do is have your doctor write out a lab order form, then you take this form to the nearest Theranos Wellness Center, which are located in Walgreens. A Walgreens' technician will take and process your blood. Once the blood has been processed, Theranos states that you can view your results via your smartphone through the Theranos mobile app. As you can see in the chart below, the cost of Theranos' blood testing is considerably less than what you might pay for blood testing work that is done through a company like Quest Diagnostics. However, before you run out to find your nearest Theranos location, Theranos is only offered in Arizona and California. However, Theranos' website states that more locations are on the way.

theran⊙s

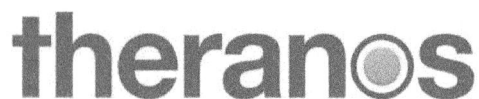

Cost for Theranos' services		
Blood test	Contents	Cost*
Basic Health for Men	Complete Blood Count, Metabolic panel, Hemoglobin A1C, Lipid panel, Prostate Specific Antigen, Thyroid Stimulating Hormone, Urinalysis complete	$54.88
Basic Health for Women	Complete Blood Count, Metabolic panel, Hemoglobin A1C, Lipid panel, Thyroid Stimulating Hormone, Urinalysis complete	$42.23
Lipid Panel	Lipid Panel; Coronary Risk Panel	$9.21
Low Density Lipoprotein	Direct LDL-C; Direct LDL; DLDL; LDL D	$6.56
High Density Lipoprotein	HDL; HDL-C	$5.63
Glucose	Blood Sugar; Fasting Blood Sugar; FBS; Fasting Blood Glucose; FBG; Blood Glucose	$2.70
Testosterone, Total	Total Testosterone	$17.75

There's an app for that!

When you get the results of your blood work back, don't worry if you don't know what Creatinine, BUN and A1C stand for. Since none of us truly know what all the acronyms mean, the American Association of Clinical Chemistry and Nika Informatics have developed apps and a website to help us to understand just what all of these acronyms mean. The Quick LabRef app is free and the Lab Tests Online app is currently $.99. Both apps work with either an IPhone or an Android smartphone. A link to these websites are located in the resources section of this book.

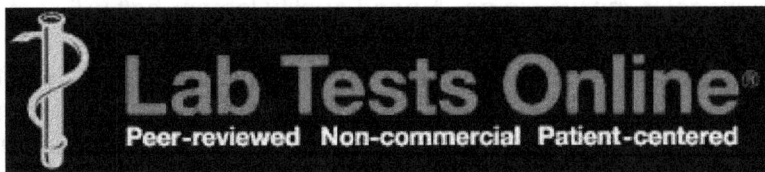

Get the proper exercise equipment.

Weight lifting belt

For those who chose to incorporate squats, deadlifts, bent over rows, snatches, or heavy lunges into their exercise plans, I highly recommend that you purchase and use a good quality weightlifting belt. I can recall a time when I was on my third set of squats at a Gold's Gym in Colorado and failed to realize that the smith machine that I was using, was stuck. Unknowingly, I was not only pushing against the weight, but I was also pushing against the weight of the entire machine which was bolted to the floor. I eventually lost that battle and had to be carried out of the gym and into my car. The only thing that saved my back was my sturdy weightlifting belt. I suffered a severe muscle strain, which took me almost 8 months to recover from. That was okay with me, considering that I didn't break anything. Back injuries are the worst.

The lifting belt serves two purposes; 1) Supports and reduces stress on the spine and; 2) increases your performance. A lifting belt allows you to increase intra-abdominal pressure to create internal support for the spine, while the core muscles in the abdominal wall and lower back push on the spine from the outside. There are some people who argue that the use of a weight belt weakens the back. Trust me, there is no research to support that notion and I can verify that the use of a weightlifting belt has actually helped me to strengthen my back. In a 2006 study, it was found that wearing a tight and stiff back belt while inhaling before lifting reduces spine load.[55] During a heavy movement like a squat, you take a deep breath, which creates the intra-abdominal pressure and then you hold this breath during the movement. This is called the Valsalva Maneuver. I know that as trainers, ACSM discourages the use of the Valsalva Maneuver, due to the significant increase in blood pressure, however there is a way to ensure that you perform this maneuver safely.

I've used nylon belts, thin leather belts, and belts that have a broader width in the middle of the belt. The best belts that I've come across are leather/suede belts that are 4 inches in width throughout the entire length of the belt and at least a half an inch thick. There are certainly more dainty looking weight belts on the market, but if you value your back, the 4-inch model is the way to go. A good quality leather belt will cost anywhere from $30 to $200 (special order).

In one study, research showed that the use of a weight belt increased the lifter's explosive power by increasing the speed of the movement without compromising the joint range of motion or overall lifting technique.[55] Another study demonstrated that wearing a lifting belt during squats increased the muscle activity of the quadriceps and hamstrings muscles. In other words, wearing a lifting belt will not only help you to lift safely, but will also increase your lifting performance.

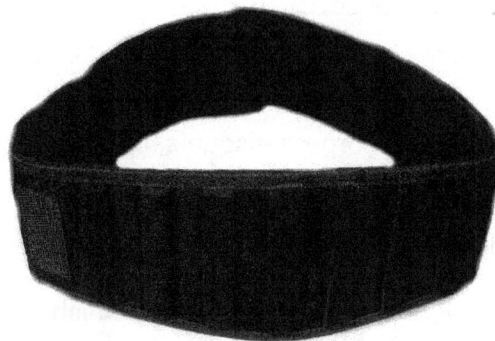

Soft neoprene lifting belt (Good)

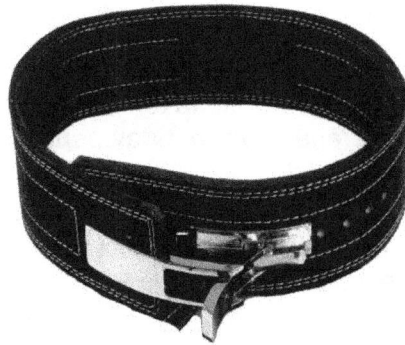

Sturdy leather lifting belt (Best)

Heart rate monitor

If you don't know by now, a heart rate monitor (HRM) is an essential piece of equipment for any weight loss, circuit training or cardiovascular program. During physical activity you will need to monitor your heart rate to ensure that you apply the proper intensity to your exercises. HRM's have been around since the 1980's. The price of monitors can range from as little as $12 to several hundred dollars. How much you spend on a HRM will dictate what features the HRM will have. Some HRM's have the following features:

- Global positioning system (GPS)-this feature is typically used to determine where and how far you've run, walked or biked.
- Calories burned-The number of calories that you burn is an estimate that is calculated using several factors to include your age, gender, and weight.
- Lap timer/splits-This feature is useful for those who typically run multiple distances shorter than 1 to 2 miles, at one time.
- Ant+ technology-allows data to be shared between the HRM and smartphones and computers.
- Water resistant/Waterproof-Some HRMs are water resistant up to 200 ft. and some are completely waterproof. Waterproof models are designed for swimmers.
- Alarm
- Rechargeable
- Trainer
- Bluetooth

Typical Heart rate measurements	
Resting heart rate HR_{rest}	Your heart rate taken first thing in the morning, at rest and averaged over a 3-day period.
Maximal Heart $Rate_{max}$	Your heart rate at an all-out effort commonly estimated by subtracting your age from 220 bpm.
Training Heart Rate (THR)	A heart rate range created to allow you to train at a specific intensity level.
Heart Rate Reserve (HRR)	The difference between maximum and resting heart rates.
Recovery Heart Rate	Reflects the rate at which the heart recovers from exercise.

Monitors can be worn on the wrist or some utilize a chest strap along with a wrist worn monitor. Heart rate monitors can be used to measure your resting heart rate, maximal heart rate, training heart rate, heart rate reserve and recovery heart rate. I found that the chest strap works best simply because of its location and its constant contact with the skin. I also found that wrist worn monitors have difficulty staying in contact with the skin.

Body composition measurement devices

Understanding your body composition and the distribution of body fat, bone mass and muscle mass within your body is a cornerstone to developing a comprehensive health and fitness program. A body composed of a high percentage of fat as compared to muscle mass, has a higher risk of certain diseases such as hypertension, diabetes, increased serum cholesterol and ultimately increased mortality. A body with a skeletal structure having low bone density has a higher risk of osteoporosis, falls and posture issues. There are several different methods for determining what your body composition is and inherently what your risk is for certain diseases.

Methods to measure body composition have certainly come along way. Dating back to the 1900's all the way to the 1970's, methods to determine body composition ranged from removal of a small amount of tissue from a living subject, to direct chemical analysis and analysis of cadavers. Fast forward to today, we have a variety of methods to choose from. Some methods are more accurate, cost effective and readily available than others.

There are two different methods for determining body composition, reference methods and prediction methods. Reference methods directly measure a component or components of the body and body fat percentage is then determined. A prediction method indirectly measures a component or components which are then compared to a reference method that predicts the same value of a reference method. Some examples of reference methods are underwater weighing, often called hydrostatic weighing, Dual energy X-ray absorptiometry (DEXA) and the four component method.[32] Prediction methods include skinfold measurements (caliper tests), body mass index (bmi), body circumferences, bioelectric impedance and electrical impedance myography.   Body composition methods are further broken down by the number of components that the method measures. Two component methods divide the body into two parts, fat mass and fat-free mass (FFM). Three component methods divide the body into fat mass, total body water and the remaining solids (protein and minerals). A four component model consist of fat mass, total body water, protein and bone minerals.[32]

Underwater weighing (Hydrodensitometry)

Underwater weighing is probably the most commonly known method for measuring body composition. This 2 component method is often called the "gold standard" because of its widespread use. This method is based on the Archimedes principle which states that when a body is immersed in water, it is buoyed by a counterforce equal to the weight of the water displaced. Bone and muscle tissue are denser than water, whereas fat is less dense. This process involves weighing a person prior to being submerged in a tank full of water. Prior to submersion, the individual exhales all of the air out of his/her lungs and then the person is submerged and then weighed while underwater. Factors such as gender, ethnicity, bone density, age, physical activity and certain diseases can have a negative effect on the results of the test. However, some corrections can be made by incorporating various formulas, like SIRI, into the final readings. Because this method uses a very large water tank, underwater weighing is performed at colleges, universities or medical centers. There is also a portable version that houses the water tank into the rear of a truck. The cost can range from $60 to $80 for each session.

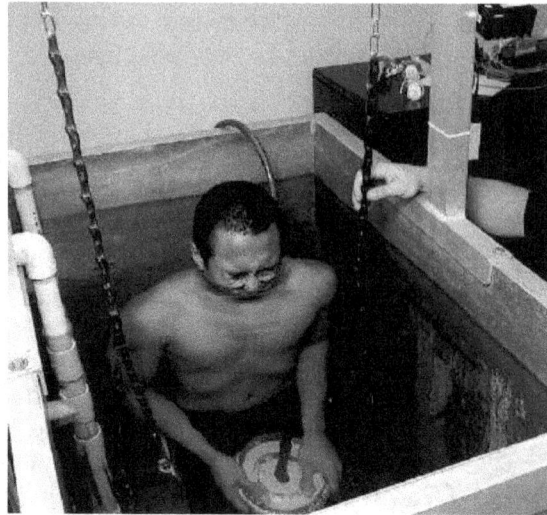

Air Displacement Plethysmography (Bodpod)

Better known as the Bodpod, this 2 component method is based on the same Archimedes principle as underwater weighing. I've actually had my body fat measurements completed in the Bodpod right before several of my competitions. The testing process required me to wear compression shorts and no shirt. If I had hair, I'd have to wear a tight fitting cap, like a swim cap. Women have to wear a Spandex like swimsuit or single layer compression shorts. The reason that you have to wear tight fitting clothes is because air can get trapped in various places throughout the body and can alter the testing results. During testing you have to sit in an egg shaped like container (More like the egg shaped capsule on the Mork and Mindy show.). A computer is linked to the testing chambers and spits out your results. This method is not suggested for kids or infants. The cost associated with this testing method runs around $45-$60 per session. Some facilities that own Bodpods, often sell packages which reduces the per session cost.

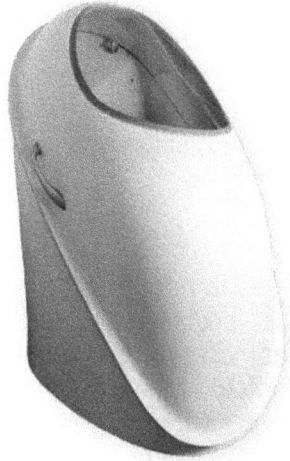

Bioelectrical impedance (BIA)

These devices can come in a scale version or a handheld version, but they both utilize the same technology. Because of the small size and low cost of the handheld version, bioelectrical impedance is widely used by fitness facilities and by individual consumers. Bioelectric impedance devices pass an alternating current through the body in order to determine the resistance of tissues. The premise behind this technology is body fat is a poor conductor and muscle mass, because it is 70% or more water, is a good conductor. Body fat (And other components) provides the resistance. This method measures your total body water and makes certain assumptions about hydration levels to determine fat percentage. There are several strict protocols that must be followed before testing with BIA. The protocols are:

- No eating or drinking within 4 hours of the test
- No exercise within 12 hours of the test
- Urinate completely within 30 minutes of the test
- No alcohol consumption in the previous 48 hours before the test

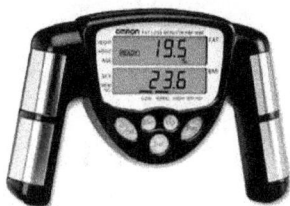

From my experience almost no one follows these protocols and most trainers that I talk to, don't even know that these protocols exist. From time to time I'll see someone jump off a BIA scale in horror after they've seen their results. Much of the horror can be avoided if the protocols listed above, are followed. Bioelectrical impedance devices can run from $30 to $8,000 for a body composition analyzer.

Skinfold calipers

Because of the skill that is needed to complete an accurate test, this method is mostly used by personal trainers and health professionals. Although calipers are fairly inexpensive it is not suggested that individual consumers attempt to utilize this method due to the fact that some of the skinfold sites are unreachable through self-analysis. This 2 component method predicts body fat percentage based on the principle that the proportion of subcutaneous fat to total fat is proportional to the total amount of body fat. However, true results vary depending on age, gender and ethnicity. This process uses several skinfold site measurements from specific locations on the body and uses the cumulative measurements to determine body fat percentage. Some skinfold methods use as little as 3 skinfold sites to up to 9 skinfold sites, in order to increase the accuracy of the results. The accuracy of this method is somewhat questionable since results can vary between two different test administrators and also by the same test administrator. Another reason is that it is hard to pinch the skin of individuals who have a significant amount of subcutaneous body fat, and some people just don't like to be touched. Test administrators aren't considered proficient until at least 150-200 skinfold assessments have been completed. Health clubs tend to include this test in personal training packages, but you can request an individual test, as a standalone service. Test can run from as little as $15 to $50 per test. If you chose to do your own testing, price ranges for skinfold calipers can run from $5 to $300, for the highest quality caliper. Metal calipers tend to produce the best results.

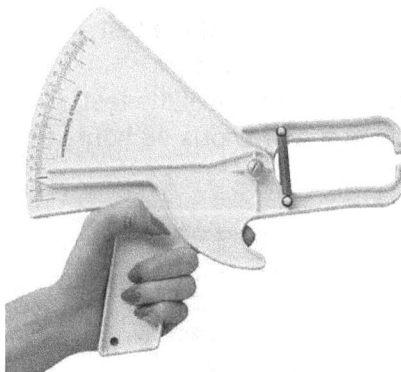

Electrical impedance myography (EIM)

Electrical impedance myography actually got its start as a non-invasive way to measure muscle deterioration in patients with disorders like muscular dystrophy, nerve injuries and Lou Gehrig's disease (ALS). If you know anything about ALS, then you know that signals from the brain progressively decline over the duration of a person's life who has ALS. When these signals decline the brain can no longer control muscle movement. Because of this lack of movement, muscles begin to atrophy. EIM can use the changes in structure and composition of the muscle to measure changes to the muscle over time. Although the technology has been around for quite some time, EIM is making an appearance as an individual consumer device.

This technology uses impedance principles like bioelectric impedance, but unlike BIA, the alternating current only passes through the muscle group that you are attempting to measure and not through your entire body. This means that this device can provide you a body fat measurement for specific muscle groups, a feature that BIA and other body composition methods can't offer. The EIM device shown in this book also offers a new measurement called muscle quality or MQ. Muscle quality measures the leanest of the muscle group being measured. Because EIM uses a localized current, EIM is not susceptible to the same issues which cause errors and inaccurate readings in BIA. An EIM consumer device costs approximately between $150 to $200.

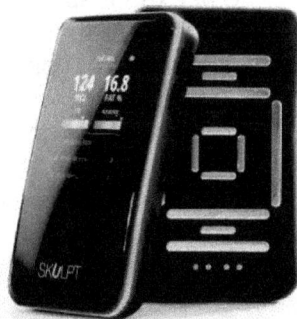

Components of physical fitness

To ensure that you develop a well-rounded exercise or training program you should develop your program around the five (5) components of physical fitness. Developing a program based on these five components ensures overall physical health. The five (5) components are listed below. [56]

Flexibility-Ensures that your joints have an acceptable range of motion. It is important that you stretch after your warm-up and after your workout to reduce injury and to help to achieve the proper range of motion. You should see an improvement in your flexibility in approximately 4 weeks of repeated stretching.

Cardiorespiratory (Aerobic)-Increases the capacity of the heart, lungs and blood carrying vessels to deliver oxygen. The goal of a good aerobic exercise program is to increase your VO2max. VO2max is simply a measure of the maximum amount of oxygen one can consume. On average, you will notice an increase in capacity (VO2max) after approximately 12 weeks of continuous aerobic exercise.

Muscular endurance-This is the muscle's ability to perform repeated contractions at sub-maximal force or to hold static contractions. Using weight that is <50% of your 1 repetition maximum (1RM) and moving that weight for more than 12 repetitions, is considered muscular endurance. These exercises utilize your Type I and some of your Type IIA muscle fibers which are smaller in size than Type IIx muscle fibers. You'll find that marathon runners are more associated with Type 1 fibers whereas sprinters are more associated with Type IIx fibers. Type I and Type IIA muscle fibers are mainly used for aerobic physical activity like endurance running, jogging and distance swimming.

Muscular strength-The amount of force a muscle can exert in a single all-out effort also called 1 rep max or 1RM. Using weight that is >70% of 1RM in a resistance training program has been shown to increase muscular strength. Repetitions should be kept between 1-12. Some muscular strength programs use weights that are >100% of 1RM. Type IIA muscle fibers are used for anaerobic physical activity such as sprinting, powerlifting and resistance training.

Body Composition-Is the ratio of lean mass compared to fat mass. Expect to see a visual change in your body composition at around 16 weeks of continuous compliance with your exercise program. However, some people have reported a change within a shorter period of time.

Note: Recent research has shown that there are at least seven types of muscle fibers, however for simplicity I've used the three most commonly known types of fibers.

Principles of training

Before you develop your cardiorespiratory and resistance training programs you should know the principles of training. These six principles should be used as a framework for developing these programs.[57]

Specificity-This principle simply states that you train your body in a specific manner to produce a specific outcome. If your goal is to lose weight, then you train in a manner that will allow you to lose weight. If your goal is to increase strength for a specific sport, then you train in a manner that will give you the added strength increase to produce a competitive advantage. In other words, simply working out with no purpose or goal in mind, is an exercise in futility.

Overload-As you move further in this chapter, you'll learn more about the word "intensity" and how it applies to physical activity and exercise. For example, in order to increase strength or increase the oxygen capacity of your lungs and heart, you will need to progressively increase the intensity of your exercises because your body will become accustomed to the intensity that is normally used. For example, if your goal is to increase the distance that you can run from 1 mile to 2 miles, you will need to overload your body to achieve this goal. Some people use high altitude training or interval training to overload their bodies to increase their running duration. This same thought process applies to resistance or anaerobic training.

Individuality-A training program should be developed based on the specific needs, goals and abilities of the person for whom it is designed. There isn't a one size fits all for exercise prescription. What works for me, may not work for the person right next to me. We are all different and those differences cannot be overlooked. Due to certain physical limitations called contraindications, there are a number of specific exercises that a person should not perform. For example, if someone has recently had problems with their knees, exercises like squats or lunges may not be the best option.

Variation-Physiologically speaking, the human body does a great job at adapting to its environment. Your body's ability to adapt to training programs is no different. When the body does adapt, a new stimulus must be imposed to further progress. Exercise and training programs should be periodized. Periodization refers to the systematic manipulation of the acute variables of training over a specific period that may range from days to years. Certain out of the box High Intensity Interval training (HITT) programs like Insanity© and PX90© are good examples of using the technique of variation and periodization to manipulate variables of a training program.

Maintenance-The great thing about starting an exercise or training program is there is light at the end of the tunnel. Once you reach your fitness goals, you merely need to maintain the level of fitness that you achieved.

Reversibility-Simply put, if you don't use it, you lose it. Any gains that you achieve in muscular strength, flexibility, muscular endurance, cardiorespiratory fitness will be lost as soon as you stop your exercise or training program.

Importance of the Warm-up

Have you ever taken a piece of gum right out of the pack and torn it in half? It's pretty easy to tear it when it's cold and dry. Now try tearing that same piece of gum after you've chewed on it for a while. You can't tear the gum like you did when it was fresh out the pack, can you? Well, your muscles act in a similar way. When your muscles are cold they are at a higher risk for tearing or being injured. During a warm-up, the blood flow to the muscles that are being worked, increases through a process called vasodilation. Your muscles will also experience an increase in the amount of oxygen and nutrients that supply the muscles that are being worked, during warm-up. Waste removal of such things as carbon dioxide and other by-products of metabolism is also increased. These events help to prevent injuries and these events also help to increase muscle performance. When your muscles are cold, reduced amounts of blood, oxygen and nutrients are channeled to muscles through a process called vasoconstriction. This is why it is important to keep your muscles warm before and during the performance of exercises. Keeping rest periods short between sets and exercises helps to keep your muscles warm, prevents injury, increases metabolism and increases muscular performance. Having extended periods of idle chit-chat during sets and exercises cools down the muscles and reduces muscular performance. A warm-up should last for at least 5-10 minutes and until a light sweat is built up.

Importance of the Cool-down

During exercise, almost 80% of the blood in a human body goes to working muscles. This means that blood to the brain and other organs is limited during exercise. Blood also pools in the legs through a condition called venous pooling. The cool down is important because it allows for a gradual return of blood to the brain and other organs which helps to prevent dizziness or even fainting. A cool-down should last for at least 5 to 10 minutes.

Stages of conditioning

Initial

The initial stage of an exercise program typically lasts several weeks. This stage is used to prepare the body for more strenuous exercise, prior to advancing to the next stage of conditioning.

Improvement

The improvement stage lasts for about 4-8 months, but can last longer, depending on the specific purpose of the training program. Some Olympic athletes may stay in this stage for over a year or more. The intensity level of the training program is increased well above the intensity levels reached during the initial stage. The improvement stage lasts until specific goals are reached. Once these goals are reached, the improvement stage is no longer needed.

Maintenance

The maintenance stage is meant to help to maintain the goals that were reached during the improvement stage. Use of a variety of physical fitness activities can be used during this stage. This stage lasts until new goals are added to an exercise program. Once new goals are added then conditioning starts at the initial stage.

Types of cardiorespiratory (aerobic) programs

Steady State

Steady state exercises include the treadmill, the stair stepper, or the stationary bicycle. These types of exercises are great for the beginner to intermediate exerciser. Because of its repetitive and unexciting nature these types of exercises can become mundane and boring. However, you can spruce up these types of exercises by varying the intensity and frequency of these exercises, as is done in AIT.

Aerobic Interval Training (AIT)

AIT can use the same type exercises as in Steady State. However, short intense burst of exercise is used intermittently throughout the duration of the workout. You'll find that AIT offers more fat burning ability than steady state exercises. An example of AIT, is running sprints while on a treadmill and adjusting the incline to raise the intensity of the exercise. You'll find that on average, your heart rate reaches higher levels than in a steady state exercise.

Anaerobic Interval Training (ANI)

Most people know ANI by the acronym HIIT or High Intensity Interval Training. HIIT uses short, intense bouts of anaerobic exercise with passive bouts of recovery. Tabata, Bibala and Timmons type training falls within this category. Tabata exercises reach workloads at or above 100% of VO2max. Gibala exercises can reach workloads of at least 95% of VO2max.

Multimode Training

If you are tired of just walking or running on a treadmill, you can mix it up a bit with multimode training. For example, you can complete 10 minutes of exercise on a stationary bicycle and then jump on the elliptical for another 10 minutes. For each of these exercises, you can incorporate AIT by keeping a steady pace for 1 minute and then work towards 100% VO2max during the subsequent minute. You can alternate the pace each minute for the entire 10-minute duration.

Stepwise or Pyramid Training

This type of training can be used for aerobic and anaerobic exercise programs. Pyramid training involves incremental increases and/or decreases in the load or resistance that is placed on the body. For example, in an aerobic program, while using the treadmill, you can gradually increase the speed of the treadmill in increments of 1-2 miles per hour during the warm-up phase all the way to the conditioning phase. In an anaerobic program, such as a resistance program you can use the same amount of weight during each set, but the number of repetitions for each set can be dropped. For example, you might start with 10 repetitions for the 1st set and then drop the number of repetitions by one, for each subsequent set. (10, 9, 8, 7, 6 and so on.)

Mixed Tempo, Undulating, or Fartlek Training

This type of training predates the 1940's which blends continuous training with interval training. Fartlek which means "speed play" in Swedish incorporates periods of fast running intermixed with periods of slower running. For beginners a person might incorporate walking and jogging together during the duration of the exercise program. For those who are more advanced, a person might alternate between sprinting and jogging.

Split Routine Training

This type of training splits your aerobic exercise session into multiple sessions. For example, if your goal is to complete 20 minutes of cardio, you can split the 20 minutes into two 10-minute aerobic exercise sessions.

How your body responds to aerobic exercise.

I can't stress enough how important aerobic exercise is to your overall health. Participating in a regular aerobic exercise program improves the functionality of your heart, blood vessels and lungs. Aerobic activity also helps you to lose weight, reduce your blood pressure and increase insulin sensitivity. During aerobic activity your body responds in an amazing way. For starters, your heart rate increases in response to the added workload, pushing more blood to the muscle groups being exercised. Since we only have so much blood in our body (approx. 5 liters), less blood is pumped to the brain when exercising which may cause dizziness or faintness. This event is called venous pooling. So it is extremely important that you take 5-10 minutes to cool down after an aerobic workout to prevent from feeling dizzy or fainting. Not only does your heart rate increase but so does the amount of blood that is pumped from the left ventricle of your heart. Your blood pressure increases and so does the amount of oxygen that your body consumes. The long term effect of these aerobic events result in a lower resting heart rate, lower blood pressure and a reduction in blood lactate. Additionally, aerobic activity uses more calories than anaerobic activity, causing you to burn more body fat. Aerobic activity includes running, cross country skiing, walking, spinning, cardio machines (treadmill, elliptical, stair stepper, arm ergometry, and aerobic classes) and some types of body weight exercises.

So what is a normal heart rate?

A healthy heart beats between 60 to 100 bpm while at rest. If your resting heart rate is higher than 100 bpm, then you may have a condition called tachycardia. If your resting heart rate is less than 60 bpm, then you may have a condition called brachycardia. Because the heart is beating so slow, some may feel fatigued, dizzy and some may even faint. However, people who consistently meet or exceed the American College of Sports Medicine's recommendations for aerobic training and resistance training may have an athletic heart syndrome. It is not uncommon for people with this syndrome to see their heart rate drop between 40-50 bpm. I've experienced a resting heart rate of 40-45 bpm after performing strenuous aerobic exercises over a several month period. Consult with your primary care physician or other health professional to determine if you have a healthy, normal heart rate.

You don't always have to exercise to burn calories. (NEAT)

Non-Exercise Activity Thermogenesis or NEAT has demonstrated that calories can be burned throughout the day from normal daily activities. In an article published in the Mayo Clinic's Endocrinology Update, Dr. James Levine asserts that the role of NEAT is more important than we think.[58] NEAT is energy expended from activities that do not include sleeping, eating or exercise. Activities like walking further than normal to the restroom, typing or cutting the grass can increase the metabolic rate, thereby burning more calories. Dr. Levine's research demonstrated that culture plays a role in the existence of NEAT. People who work in agricultural or manual labor type jobs have high NEAT, whereas wealth and industrialization appear to decrease NEAT. Dr. Levine further breaks down NEAT into two categories; Occupational NEAT and Leisure NEAT. He compares a sedentary occupation to a strenuous work occupation like farming and shows that a strenuous occupation can burn at least a 2,000 calories more than a chair bound occupation, where moving is limited. Leisure activities can vary too. Watching television may burn 30 calories as compared to 600 calories for leisure activities like gardening and home repair.

So what can you do? If you have a sedentary like desk job, you should get up from the desk and take a brisk walk down the hall or around the office, every few hours. Instead of watching television for several hours, you can pursue a home improvement project, garden or do additional chores around the house. Even if you feel the need to watch your favorite television show, you can get up during each commercial break, walk around and be ready when the commercial break is over. However, a word of caution. Snacking while watching television, only adds more calories to the number of calories that are needed to lose weight.

How to develop your own aerobic exercise program.

Generally speaking, the goal of a weight loss program is not just to lose weight, it's to change your body composition. As we know as our body composition changes body weight may or may not change. We've heard the stories about people expressing concern that the amount of weight that they have lost hasn't changed, but the clothes that they used to wear no longer fit. This phenomenon occurs because their body composition has changed. Remember, a pound of body fat takes up 25% more space than a pound of muscle.

The strategy of an exercise program developed for weight loss is to:

- Reduce body fat-Reduces your risk for certain diseases.
- Gain muscle-Increases your metabolism, reduces bone and muscle loss.
- Create an energy deficit-increases the amount of calories burned.

A weight loss program should include aerobic activity to burn body fat and resistance training to build muscle and increase bone density. A weight loss program should be created based on ACSM's and NASM's framework represented by the acronym F.I.T.T.E.[59] as shown below.

- **Frequency**-Engage in cardiorespiratory exercises 3-5 days per week.

- **Intensity**-For beginners or those who have been sedentary 30% of heart rate reserve (HRR) and up to 85% of HRR for conditioned individuals.

- **Time/Duration**-cardiorespiratory exercises should last between 20-90 minutes however 10 minute intermittent exercises which add up to 20-90 should suffice.

- **Type/mode**-The type of cardiorespiratory exercises that an individual performs should be tailored to the individual. For example, if someone has knee problems, an arm ergometer should be the best option for an aerobic exercise. Studies have shown that an arm ergometer can be as good as running on a treadmill.

- **Enjoyment**-No one stays committed to doing things that they don't like to do. A program should attempt to incorporate as many positive and rewarding experiences as possible. For example, some people thoroughly enjoy exercising outdoors instead of exercising in a gym.

Note: The following pages outline the method of developing a basic exercise plan. In order to develop a more advanced exercise plan, it is suggested to use a certified health/exercise professional who is credentialed by an accredited certifying agency. To verify if a health/exercise professional is certified through an accredited certifying agency, go to the resources section of this book and use the link for the United States Registry of Exercise Professionals.

Now let's follow Marilyn as she develops her cardiorespiratory (aerobic) program.

Step 1-As mentioned earlier in this chapter, take a health assessment prior to developing an exercise program. Again, a typical health assessment consists of a health questionnaire, lipid and metabolic panels. As mentioned previously, Marilyn went through a thorough health assessment which included a questionnaire, metabolic panel and lipid panel. It was determined that Marilyn can perform most types of exercises without incorporating any restrictions.

Step 2-Determine what your resting heart rate is. Your resting heart rate will be used in Step 3 of the development of an aerobic program. Measure your resting heart rate when you wake up in the morning and before you get out of bed. Place your index and middle fingers from either hand and place them on your radial (wrist with your palm faced up) artery. Count how many beats you can feel within 60 seconds. You can use a stopwatch to determine when 60 seconds has lapsed. Repeat this for three days and average the three measurements. This will be your resting heart rate. (A link to a how to video is included on the resources page at the end of this book.)

Over a period of three mornings, Marilyn used the stopwatch on her smartphone to measure her resting heart rate. Her three measurements were 56 bpm, 54 bpm, and 56 bpm. Her average resting heart rate is 55 bpm.

Step 3.-Determine what your Heart Rate Reserve (HRR*) is. Follow the example below.

Formula

220-your age=HRmax

HRmax-resting heart rate=HRR

(HRR x Intensity) + resting heart rate=

Example: Marilyn is a 35-year-old previously sedentary individual with a resting heart rate of 55 bpm.

220-35(age)=185 bpm (HRmax)

185 bpm-55(resting heart rate) =130 bpm
(130 x 30%*) +55 bpm= 94 bpm (HRR)

Step 4.-Determine your frequency and intensity. (see chart on next page).

*Since Marilyn has been sedentary for the last 6 months, she has determined that during her initial phase of her program, her exercise intensity will be 30% of HRR and the duration of her aerobic exercise will last for at least 20 minutes.

Step 5.-Use a heart rate monitor to determine if you've reached and maintained your HRR during the entire duration of your aerobic activities.

Marilyn purchased a heart rate monitor to ensure that she maintains 94 bpm, throughout the entire duration of her workout. Marilyn's entire aerobic exercise plan is displayed on the next page.

*Heart Rate Reserve (HRR)- is the difference between a person's measured or predicted maximum heart rate and resting heart rate. HRR is used instead of HRmax because the measurements are more tailored to your specific fitness level. HRmax simply subtracts your age from 220, which as we know not everyone who has the same age is at the same fitness level. So HRR is a better more tailored measure than HRmax

Marilyn's cardiorespiratory (aerobic) program

Phase	Week	Frequency (per week)	Intensity (% x HRR)	Time** (minutes)	Type	Marilyn's target heart rate during exercise (bpm)***
Initial	1	3*	30%	20**	Brisk walk outdoors	94
	2	3	35%	20	Treadmill	100.5
	3	3	35%	20	Elliptical	100.5
	4	3	40%	20	Bicycle	107
Improvement	5-8	3-4	45%-50%	25	Recumbent Bicycle	113.5-120
	9-12	3-4	50%-60%	30	Treadmill	120-133

	13-16	4-5	50%-70%	30-40	Run outdoors	120-146
	17-20	4-5	55%-85%	30-40	Elliptical	126.5-165.5
	21-26	4-5	70%-85%	30-40	Bicycle	146-165.5
Maintenance	27+	3-4	70%-85%	30-40	Recumbent Bicycle	146-165.5

*-For those who are classified as being significantly over normal weight, frequency should be increased to 5-7 days per week.

**-During the initial phase, the time or duration can be broken out into 2 10-minute bouts of aerobic activity.

***-As Marilyn's aerobic capacity increases her resting heart rate will decline. This means that she should reassess her resting heart rate and recalculate her HRR in weeks 4, 13, 21 and 27.

You should always warm-up for approximately 5-6 minutes, until you build-up a light sweat. A 5-10-minute cool down, should always follow your workouts. This prevents venous pooling as mentioned earlier in this chapter.

Types of resistance training programs.

Resistance training offers a plethora of benefits. As we age, the amount of muscle tissue that we have starts to decline. Resistance training can help to halt or reverse this process by aiding the process of muscle building. Increased muscle mass can also prevent the onset of osteoporosis and can decrease the risk of heart disease by lowering body fat, decreasing blood pressure, improving cholesterol and increasing metabolism. With all of these benefits you would think that everyone would incorporate a resistance training program into their exercise regimen. However, this is not the case. Studies have shown that only 20% of women in the United States incorporate a resistance training program into their exercise regimen. Unfortunately, this is somewhat ironic since women, on average, need resistance training more than men. Men on average have more muscle mass than women which equates to a much lower risk of diseases like osteoporosis. Women tend to spend more time in aerobic type programs like Zumba, running, Spin, Step or other cardiorespiratory activities. Men on the other hand spend most of their time performing resistance exercises and not enough aerobic exercises.

Body weight

The most traditional and well known body weight exercise is the push-up. However, using your body for resistance training has morphed into an expanded repertoire of exercises that use varying angles and positions to change the resistance and the muscle group that is worked. Body weight exercises represent the simplest and cheapest form of resistance training. Unfortunately, unless you gain weight, your body will eventually adapt to the amount of resistance that can be exerted on the muscles and strength gains will eventually plateau.

Resistance bands

A cost effective and versatile form of resistance equipment is the resistance band. A full set of resistance bands with resistance varying from 2 pounds to well over 200 pounds can be purchased for a price of $5 to $50. Resistance bands can be used inside the home, outside the home and at the gym. Because of the low cost and versatility that resistance bands offer, resistance bands can appeal to almost any budget and can fit almost any resistance program. Resistance bands are also lightweight which means they can be carried in a gym bag or even a small pocketbook. As demonstrated later in this chapter, resistance bands can be used to strengthen all the major muscle groups.

Free weights

Free weights can come in a variety of weights, colors, textures, shapes and materials. Free weights include medicine balls, kettle bells, dumbbells and sandbags. Free weights can be used in a variety of ways that selectorized weight machines cannot. Free weights are not restricted to a specific range of motion like selectorized weight machines are. The most expensive free weights tend to be metal (mainly steel) covered in rubber, while the least expensive form of free weights can be medicine balls or kettlebells. Free weights can be purchased at almost any discount department store. I've seen some great deals on free weights in the classified sections of newspapers, Craigslist and stores that specialize in refurbished or used fitness equipment.

Selectorized weight machines

Selectorized weight machines are the most expensive form of resistance equipment. You'll typically find selectorized weight machines at your local gym, college fitness facility or physical therapy office. A standalone machine, such as a leg extension machine can cost a few hundred dollars to several thousand dollars. A multi-station selectorized machine which may include a leg extension station, lateral pulldown station, and chest press station can cost upwards of $8,000 depending on the manufacturer. This type of machine does offer some benefits over free weights. To adjust the resistance on these machines, all you need to do is to place a pin into the slot that is designated for the weight that you want. However, selectorized machines must follow a defined plane and range of motion, which free weights do not. Selectorized machines can also use pneumatics for resistance instead of a weight stack.

How your body responds to resistance training

The benefits that can be received from resistance training are numerous. Resistance training helps us to fight the effects of sarcopenia and osteoporosis. Resistance training can also help to reduce the risk of heart disease by lowering body fat, decreases blood pressure, improves cholesterol and helps to provide strength and stability around our joints.

Resistance training can help to improve muscular strength and muscular endurance. Increasing muscular strength through resistance training is a gradual process. Within the first several weeks of performing resistance type exercises you will notice an increase in strength. However, the increase in strength is mainly caused by neuromuscular adaptation rather than from an increase in muscle size. Strength gains from an increase in muscle size typically won't occur for several months. Neuromuscular adaptation is the result of an increase in the communication between your brain and your muscle fibers. As communication increases between your brain and your muscle fibers, the number of muscle fibers that are used in a particular movement increases, thereby increasing your strength. Eventually as the size of your muscles increase (hypertrophy), so does your muscular strength. As you gain muscle size, the number of muscle fibers does not grow. The number of muscle fibers that you have is fixed before adolescence (girls 15-21 years; boys 18-22 years). On average muscular strength peaks in the mid-20s for both sexes and remains fairly stable through 33-37 years of age. Unfortunately, muscle strength begins to decline by 15% per decade after reaching 50 years, then 60 years, and 70 years. After 70 years, muscle strength declines by 30% per decade, thereafter. It is important to note that sedentary individuals lose 20%-40% of their muscle mass over the course of adulthood. However, you can slow down these processes by incorporating a well thought out resistance training program into your overall fitness program.

PLANES OF MOTION

There are three planes of motion; the sagittal plane, the frontal plane and the transverse plane. Why is knowing the planes of motion important to resistance training? Because your body doesn't just move in one direction. Your body can move in multiple directions, so it's important for you to strengthen all your muscles equitably. Knowing the planes of motion is even more important for those who are training for specific sports, so that specific muscles that are mainly used for competition can be strengthened and made flexible to ensure proper range of motion.

Sagittal plane

The sagittal plane divides the body into half, vertically, creating a right and left side.[1] Exercises like squats, curls, tricep extensions, leg curls, and leg extensions, help to strengthen muscles that are used for running, biking, jumping and rowing.

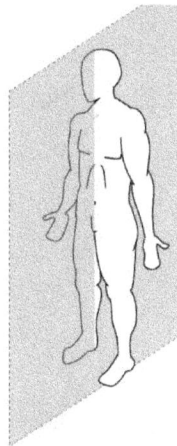

Frontal Plane

The frontal plane divides the body into half, vertically creating a front (anterior) and back (posterior).[1]

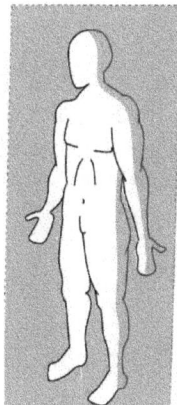

Exercises like the side lunge, adductor/abductor machines (or cables), speed skaters, military shoulder press, lateral raise, upright rows, or side lying leg lifts work muscles in the frontal plane. These exercises can be used to strengthen muscles that help to move the body side to side (laterally). Sports like baseball, basketball, tennis, and hockey depend on good and quick lateral movements.

Transverse plane

The transverse plane divides the body, horizontally, creating an upper half (superior) and lower half (inferior).[1]

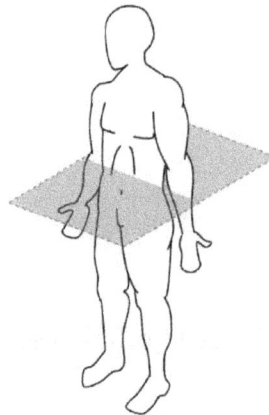

Exercises like the Russian twist, rotating one-arm cable, rotational medicine ball throw, one arm dumbbell bench press, three-point dumbbell row work muscles in the transverse plane. These exercises can be used to strengthen muscles that help to rotate the body. Sports like tennis, baseball, badminton, ping pong and even javelin throwing rely heavily on the ability of the body to rotate.

MUSCLE ACTIONS

There are three basic muscle actions; Concentric, Eccentric and isometric

Concentric muscle action

A concentric muscle action involves shortening of the muscle. This action occurs when the force exceeds the external resistance, resulting in joint movement.[57] A typical exercise that demonstrates a concentric muscle action is a single arm dumbbell curl. In the start of the movement, the arm is extended and as the force exceeds the weight of the dumbbell, the muscle shortens and the dumbbell is curled. Repeated contractions causes blood to flow into the muscles that are worked causing the muscles to feel a "pump'.

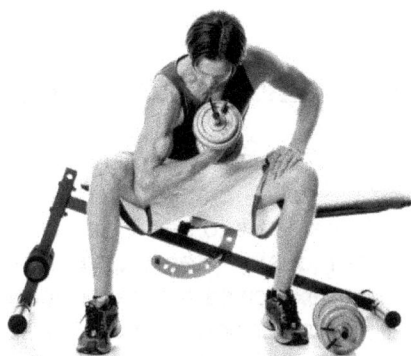

Concentric muscle action

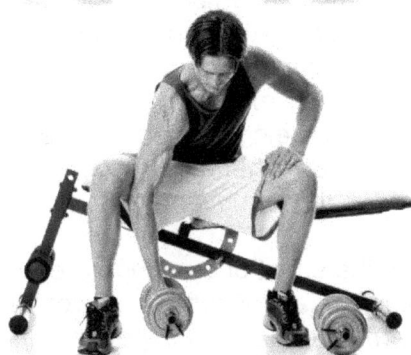

Eccentric muscle action

Eccentric muscle action

An eccentric muscle action involves lengthening of the muscle.[57] This action occurs when the external resistance exceeds the force given by the muscle. An example of an eccentric muscle action is when the dumbbell is being lowered during a bicep curl. This muscle action is often called a "negative". A muscle can generate more force during an eccentric muscle action than in a concentric muscle action. Because more force can be generated during this type of muscle action, I use this muscle action the most to increase muscle mass.

Isometric muscle action

In an isometric muscle action, the muscle neither shortens or lengthens, but still generates force. An isometric muscle action occurs when the external resistance is too heavy to move and the force supplied by the muscle is not enough to move the external resistance.[57] A good example of an isometric muscle action is to push against an object that you know weighs significantly more than your one repetition maximums. A muscle can generate more force during an isometric muscle action than in a concentric muscle action. Strength gains can be achieved from isometric muscle actions, however the strength gains are mainly static and do not appear throughout the entire range of motion.

How to develop your own basic resistance training program.

Step 1-Determine your suitability for specific exercises. Prior to starting any resistance training program, you should determine what exercises that you can or cannot perform. One important step that you should certainly consider is to see a doctor prior to starting any exercise program. In the health and fitness industry, preexisting injuries or medical issues that prevent you from performing specific exercises are called, contraindications. Some exercises can be modified to suit your particular needs. For example, a person with a past knee injury with limited range of movement may not need to go below parallel for a squat, when slightly above parallel will suffice. Additionally, some exercises may require you to develop synergistic muscles to help perform the movement and to ensure your body is within the correct plane of motion. For example, when performing the squat or the lunge the major (primary) muscles that are being worked are the quadriceps, hamstrings and gluteus maximus (butt). However, other muscles, call synergistic or stabilizers help the primary muscles to perform these movements.

The synergistic muscles that are used in the squat or the lunge are the Gluteus medius/minimus (abductors), adductors, soleus/gastrocnemius (calves), erector spinae (lower back) and transverse abdominus. Some people may experience pain in their knees, called patella-femoral pain, when performing the squat or lunge.[60] Others may notice that their knees move laterally (side to side) when performing the squat. These issues are mainly caused by overactive or underactive muscles. A muscle on the inside (Vastus medialis) or outside (Vastus Lateralis) of the upper leg could cause the knee to misalign during the squat movement which causes pain. In order to help to resolve or minimize this issue, strengthening the synergistic abductor and adductor muscles can be the fix. It is important to note that many young female athletes unfortunately suffer from patella femoral pain due to weakness in these synergistic muscles.

110

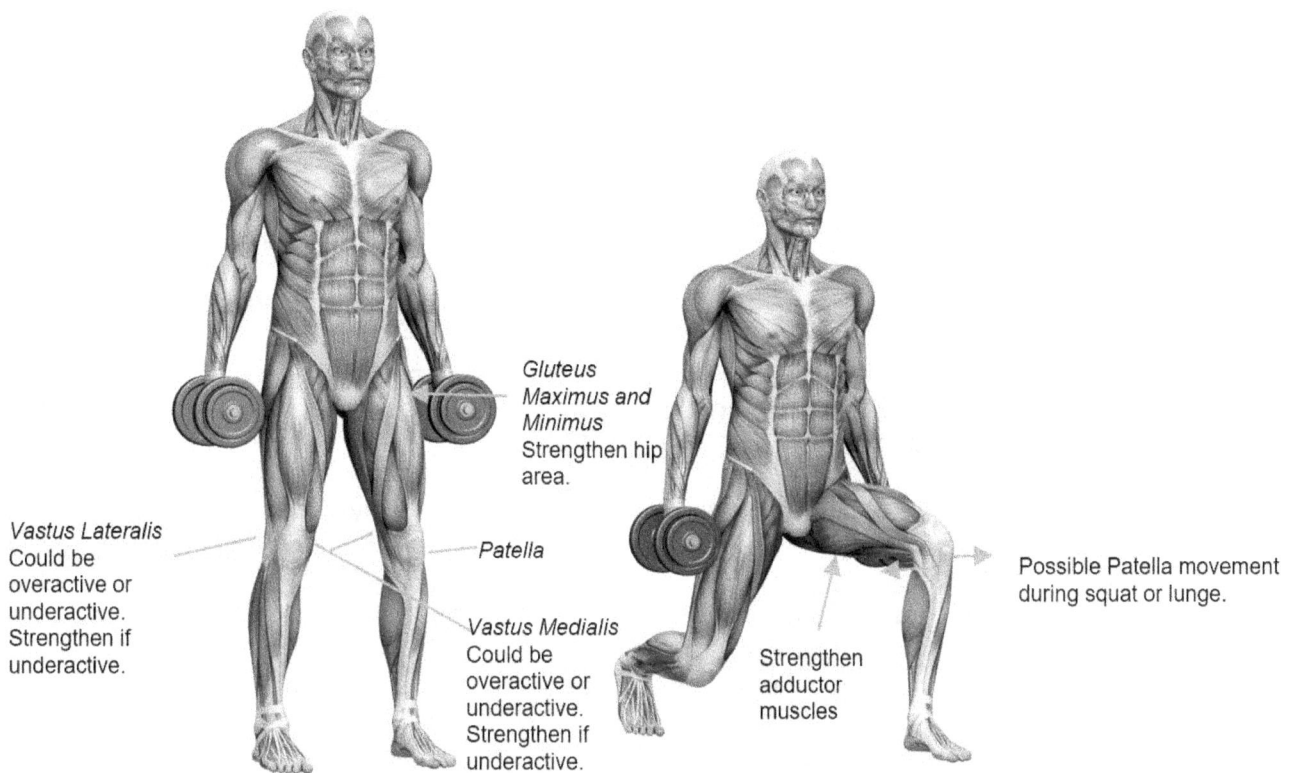

Gluteus Maximus and Minimus Strengthen hip area.

Vastus Lateralis Could be overactive or underactive. Strengthen if underactive.

Patella

Vastus Medialis Could be overactive or underactive. Strengthen if underactive.

Strengthen adductor muscles

Possible Patella movement during squat or lunge.

Step 2-Determine what type of resistance training program that you will need, based on the principle of specificity.

As previously discussed, one of the principles of resistance training is specificity. This means that a resistance training program should be developed based on a specific purpose. For example, if your goal is to gain muscle, then a resistance training program should be developed to help you to accomplish this goal. Athletes can develop a resistance training program that is tailored to help them to improve their athletic performance. The basic resistance training programs that follows, can be used for a total body workout (weight loss), 3-day split program, circuit training or for muscle building. A resistance training program is also included for those who do not have access to a health club or who prefer to workout at home or outdoors, using resistance bands.

Resistance training programs can be created for:
- Injury recovery
- Muscle Building
- Improving athletic performance

- Weight loss
- Increasing bone density
- Weight gain
- Increasing muscular endurance
- Increasing strength
- Increasing power

Step 3-Determine what your 1 repetition maximum is for each exercise that works each major muscle group. As an example, the next page shows all the 1 repetition maximums for Marilyn. Marilyn will use these numbers to help build her resistance training program.

There are several methods that can be used to determine a 1-repetition maximum. The first method can be performed in a gym or at home. Since maximum weight will be used, you will need a spotter.

- Determine what muscle group and exercise that you will use for testing. For example, if you want to determine a 1-repetition maximum for biceps, you can use a dumbbell.
- Prior to testing, ensure that a 5-6-minute warm-up is completed.
- Rest for a maximum of 1 minute
- Select the weight that allows you to complete 3-5 repetitions until you are fatigued.
- Rest for 2 minutes
- Determine the maximum weight that can be moved during the entire range of motion, for 1 repetition. Complete at least 2-3 repetitions until fatigue.
- Rest for 2 minutes
- Increase the weight, until only 1 repetition can be completed.

There are other methods such as formulas that can be used to determine a 1 repetition maximum.

Epley Formula

$1RM = w(1 + r/30)$ w=weight, r=repetitions Example: $1RM = 50lbs (1 + 6$ repetitions/30) $= 60lbs$ is the 1 repetition maximum

Lander Formula

$1RM = 110*w/101.3 - 2.67123*r$

Step 4-Based on what Marilyn determined her goal was in Step 1, she will now need to periodize her program. The premise behind periodization is that over time your body will adapt to the stress that you put on it body from your resistance training program. So you will need to change your program over a period of time in order to see continued progress. If you don't, strength may even decrease as a result. Periodization divides your resistance training program into cycles. This can be a little complicated, so we'll just keep it simple.

- Macrocycle-6 months to 1 year
- Mesocycle-several weeks to several months
- Microcycle-weekly

Marilyn has determined that her goal is to increase muscle mass which will help her to counter the possible effects of muscle wasting due to aging (sarcopenia). She is also concerned about the possibility of having to deal with osteoporosis since her bone density tests were not as promising as she would have like the results to be.

Since Marilyn has determined that her goal is to gain muscle mass (highlighted in green in the table below. *), Marilyn has decided to break her resistance training program out into weeks (microcycle). Since Marilyn is only interested in increasing muscle mass, she intends to keep your intensity to around 60% to 70% of her 1 repetition maximums as shown in her workouts on the following pages.

	To increase muscular endurance	To increase muscle Mass	To increase strength	To increase power	To peak	To maintain
Sets	3-5	3-5	3-5	3-5	1-3	Light physical activity
Reps per set	15-20+	8-12	2-6	2-3	1-3	Moderate physical activity
Intensity (% of 1RM)	<50%	50%-70%	70%-80%	80%-90%	90%-%100 (>100%)	Moderate physical activity
Volume	Very high	High	High	Moderate	Low	Moderate physical activity

Note: This example outlines the method of developing a basic exercise plan. In order to develop a more advanced exercise plan, it is suggested to use a certified health/exercise professional who is credentialed by an accredited certifying agency. To verify if a health/exercise professional is certified through an accredited certifying agency, go to the resources section of this book and use the link for the United States Registry of Exercise Professionals.

Exercise	Marilyn's 1 repetition maximums	Major Muscle Group worked
Flat bench press	100 lbs.	Pectoral/Chest
EZ Curl bar	35 lbs	Bicep/Forearm
One arm curl	20 lbs	Bicep/Forearm
Close grip bench press	90 lbs	Tricep/Chest
Tricep extension	35 lbs	Tricep
Decline press	110 lbs	Pectoral/Chest
Incline press	95 lbs	Pectoral/Chest
Tricep dip machine	40 lbs	Tricep
Squat	150 lbs	Quadriceps/Upper leg Glutes/Butt

Seated Hip abduction	120 lbs	Glutes/Butt/Hips
Barbell lunge	70 lbs	Quadriceps/Upper leg Glutes/Butt
Leg press	200 lbs	Quadriceps/Upper leg Glutes/Butt
Low-row pulley machine	80 lbs	Latissimus Dorsi/Back
Shoulder press	50 lbs	Deltoids/Shoulders
Ab Crunch machine	50 lbs	Rectus Abdominis/Abs
Seated Calf raise machine	100 lbs	Gastrocnemius/Calves
Seated Leg extension	60 lbs	Quadriceps/Upper leg
Leg curl	60 lbs	Biceps femoris/Hamstrings
One-arm dumbbell row	35 lbs	Latissimus Dorsi/Back
Lateral pulldown	80 lbs	Latissimus Dorsi/Back
Dumbbell kickback	30 lbs	Tricep

Major Muscle Groups

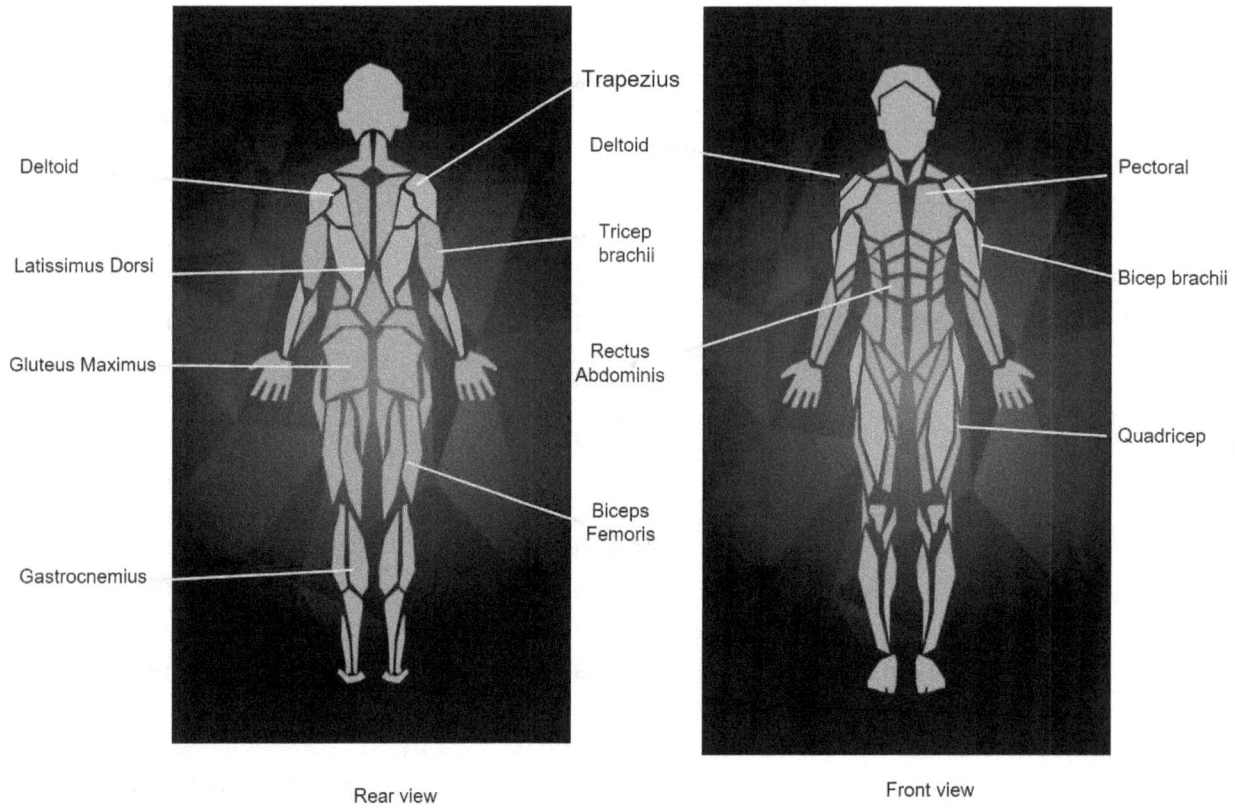

Deltoid

Latissimus Dorsi

Gluteus Maximus

Gastrocnemius

Trapezius

Deltoid

Tricep brachii

Rectus Abdominis

Biceps Femoris

Rear view

Pectoral

Bicep brachii

Quadricep

Front view

Marilyn's Workout
Week 1-2
Initial Conditioning stage

Day 1	Sets	Intensity	Reps	Day 2	Sets	Intensity	Reps	Day 3	Sets	Intensity	Reps
Warm-up		5-8 minutes		Warm-up		5-8 minutes		Warm-up		5-8 minutes	
Bench press	3	60% or 60lbs	10-12	Bench press	3	60% or 60lbs	10-12	Bench press	3	60% or 60lbs	10-12
Lateral Pulldown	3	60%or 48lbs	10-12	Lateral Pulldown	3	60%or 48lbs	10-12	Lateral Pulldown	3	60%or 48lbs	10-12
Leg Press	3	60%or 120lbs	10-12	Leg Press	3	60%or 120lbs	10-12	Leg Press	3	60%or 120lbs	10-12
Shoulder press	3	60%or 30lbs	10-12	Shoulder press	3	60%or 30lbs	10-12	Shoulder press	3	60%or 30lbs	10-12
EZ Curl Barl	3	60%or 21lbs	10-12	Dumbbell curl	3	60%or 12lbs	10-12	Dumbbell curl	3	60%or 12lbs	10-12
Tricep extension	3	60%or 21lbs	10-12	Tricep extension	3	60%or 21lbs	10-12	Tricep extension	3	60%or 21lbs	10-12
Seated calf raise	3	60%or 60lbs	12-15	Seated calf raise	3	60%or 60lbs	12-15	Seated calf raise	3	60%or 60lbs	12-15
Ab crunch	3	60%or 30lbs	15-20	Ab crunch	3	60%or 30lbs	15-20	Ab crunch	3	60%or 30lbs	15-20
Cool-down		5-8 minutes		Cool-down		5-8 minutes		Cool-down		5-8 minutes	
Stretch											

Basic Total body Resistance Program for Beginners

Marilyn's Workout
Week 1-2
Initial Conditioning stage

Day 1	Sets	Intensity	Reps	Day 2	Sets	Intensity	Reps	Day 3	Sets	Intensity	Reps
Warm-up		5-8 minutes				5-8 minutes				5-8 minutes	
Flat Bench press	3	60%or 60lbs	10-12	Squat	3	60% or 90lbs	10-12	Lateral Pulldown	3	60% or 48lbs	10-12
Incline press	3	60%x 57lbs	10-12	Leg press	3	60% or 120lbs	10-12	One-arm dumbbell row	3 x 2	60% or 21lbs	10-12
Decline press	3	60%or 66lbs	10-12	Seated leg extension	3	60% or 36lbs	10-12	Low-row pulley machine	3	60% or 48lbs	10-12
Tricep extension	3	60%or 21lbs	10-12	Seated leg curl	3	60% or 36lbs	10-12	EZ Curl Bar (standing)	3	60% or 21lbs	10-12
Tricep dip machine	3	60%x 24lbs	10-12	Barbell lunge	3	60% or 42lbs	10-12	Alternating dumbbell Hammer curl (standing)	3 x 2	60% or 12lbs	10-12
Close grip bench	3	60%x 48lbs	10-12	Seated Hip abduction	3	60% or 72lbs	10-12	Incline Alternating Dumbbell Curl	3 x 2	60% or 12lbs	10-12
Dumbbell kickback	3 x 2	60%18lbs	12-15	Seated Calf raise machine	3	60% or 60lbs	12-15	Ab Crunch	3	60%or 30lbs	20-25
Ab Crunch	3	60%or 30lbs	20-25	Russian twist	3	10lbs ball/dumbbell	15-20	Scissor Kick	3		15-20
Cool-down		5-8 minutes		Cool-down		5-8 minutes		Cool-down		5-8 minutes	
Stretch				Stretch				Stretch			

118

Marilyn's Workout
Week 3-4
Improvement conditioning phase

Day 1	Sets	Intensity	Reps	Day 2	Sets	Intensity	Reps	Day 3	Sets	Intensity	Reps
Warm-up		5-8 minutes				5-8 minutes				5-8 minutes	
Flat Bench press	3	70%or 70lbs	10-12	Squat	3	70% or 105lbs	10-12	Lateral Pulldown	3	70% or 56lbs	10-12
Incline press	3	70%x 67lbs	10-12	Leg press	3	70% or 140lbs	10-12	One-arm dumbbell row	3 x 2	70% or 25lbs	10-12
Decline press	3	70%or 77lbs	10-12	Seated leg extension	3	70% or 42lbs	10-12	Low-row pulley machine	3	70% or 56lbs	10-12
Tricep extension	3	70%or 25lbs	10-12	Seated leg curl	3	70% or 42lbs	10-12	EZ Curl Bar (standing)	3	70% or 25lbs	10-12
Tricep dip machine	3	70% or 24lbs	10-12	Barbell lunge	3	70% or 49lbs	10-12	Alternating dumbbell Hammer curl (standing)	3 x 2	70% or 14lbs	10-12
Close grip bench	3	70% or 63lb	10-12	Seated Hip abduction	3	70% or 84lbs	10-12	Incline Alternating Dumbbell Curl	3 x 2	70% or 14lbs	10-12
Dumbbell kickback	3 x 2	70% or 25lbs	12-15	Seated Calf raise machine	3	70% or 70lbs	12-15	Ab Crunch	3	70% or 35lbs	20-25
Ab crunch	3	70% or 35lbs	20-25	Russian twist	3	10lbs ball/dumbbell	15-20	Scissor Kick	3	30 secs	15-20
Cool-down		5-8 minutes		Cool-down		5-8 minutes		Cool-down		5-8 minutes	
Stretch				Stretch				Stretch			

Intermediate Total Body Resistance Program for Beginners

119

Resistance training exercises

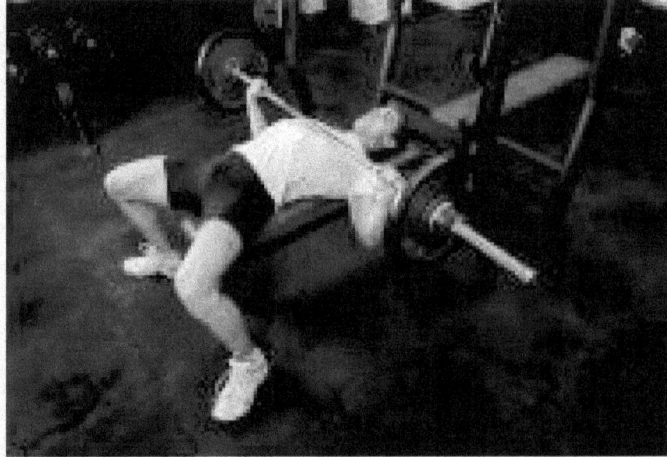

Bench Press

Major Muscles worked: Pectorals/Chest/Triceps brachii

- Keep feet flat on the floor. This is your base and helps to produce additional force.
- Grasp the bar with an overhand grip. The bar should rest just above your wrist, on the heel of your hand.
- You should lay on the blades of your shoulders. There should be a ½ inch to 1-inch space between the bench and your lower back.
- Push the bar, by bringing your elbows closer to your body. Don't by using your 7shoulders.
- The proper travel of the bar is not in a straight line from your chest, up. The proper travel is actually in a slight curve up towards your head.
- Inhale on the downward movement (eccentric) and exhale on the upward movement (concentric/contraction).
- Avoid performing the Valsava maneuver, which is to hold your breath during the entire movement. When the Valsava maneuver is performed, blood pressure rises significantly which may cause light headedness or dizziness.

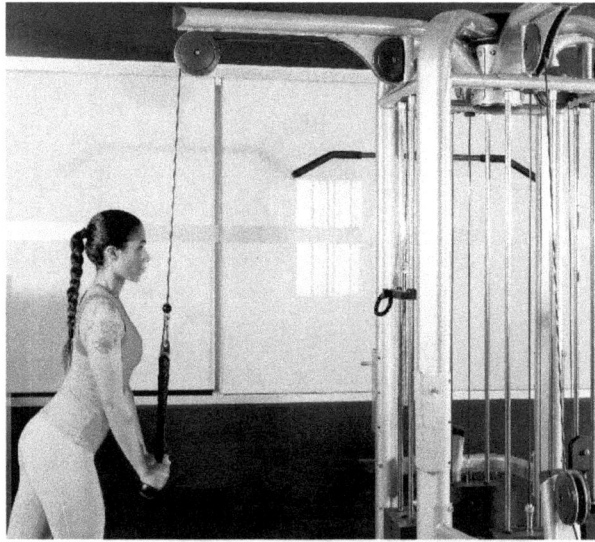

Tricep Extension

Major Muscles worked: Triceps brachii. All three heads of the tricep muscle group.

- This exercise can be performed with a rope or straight handle.
- Stand straight up while facing the cable machine.
- You should avoid leaning forward during the movement as this will engage your shoulders and lessen the work that is being done on your triceps.
- As your tricep muscles get near to exhaustion, your elbows have a tendency to move away from your body. Concentrate on keeping your elbows close to your body to ensure that your triceps are being worked and not your shoulders.
- You'll find that by doing so, the movement is harder to complete.
- Breath out during the downward movement (concentric/contraction) and breath in on the upward movement (eccentric).

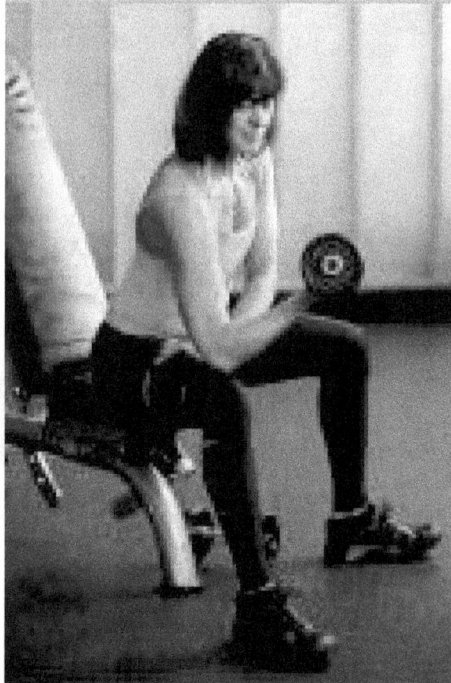

One-arm dumbbell curl

Major Muscles worked: Biceps brachii/Brachialis

- Grasp the dumbbell with an underhand grip.

- Squeeze the bicep at the top of the movement.

- Hold the dumbbell at the top of the movement and let the dumbbell down slowly, during each repetition.

- Breath out on the upward movement (concentric/contraction) and breath in on the downward movement (eccentric).

- To work the forearms and the bicep, use a hammer grip (Palm facing toward your body.)

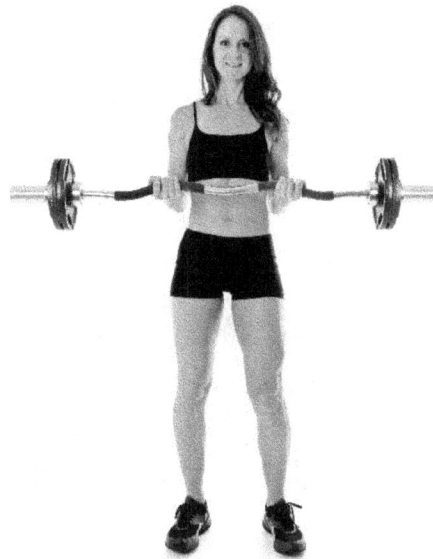

EZ-Curl bar bicep curl

Major Muscles worked: Biceps brachii/Brachialis

- Stand with your feet shoulder width apart.
- Grasp the bar with an underhand grip.
- Hold the bar at the top of the movement and let the dumbbell down slowly, during each repetition.
- Breath out on the upward movement (concentric/contraction) and breath in on the downward movement (eccentric).
- Squeeze the bicep at the top of the movement.

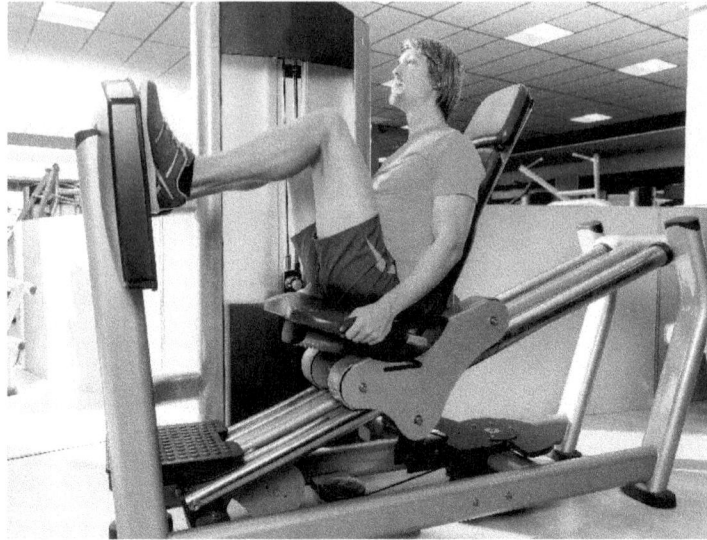

Horizontal leg press machine

Major Muscles worked: Quadriceps/Gluteus Maximus/minimus/Bicep Femoris/Soleus/Gastrocnemius

- Sit with your back up against the pad, feet shoulder width apart.

- Adjust the seat at or slightly below parallel.

- To increase the emphasis on the hamstrings, place your feet on the upper part on the foot plate.

- To increase the emphasis on calves, place the ball of your feet on the lower portion of the foot plate.

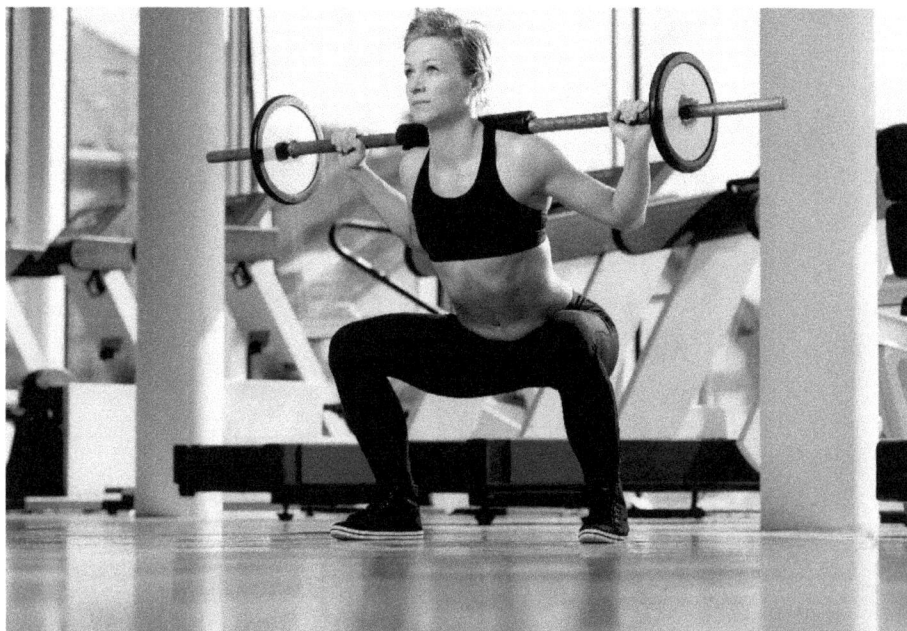

Barbell Squat

Muscles worked: Quadriceps/Gluteus Maximus-minimus/Bicep Femoris

- Use a lifting belt if lifting heavier than usual weight.
- Place the bar on the upper part of your middle back.
- Use the blocking method when squatting. This method involves taking a deep breath to fill the chest cavity and then holding your deep breath during the entire movement. This makes the rib cage rigid and prevents your upper body from leaning forward.
- Contract or squeeze your abs. This increases intra-abdominal pressure and also prevents your upper body from leaning forward.
- Contract the lower back muscles so your spinal cord is extended. This will prevent your back from rounding which may cause disc herniation.
- Squat can also be performed on a Smith machine for added safety.

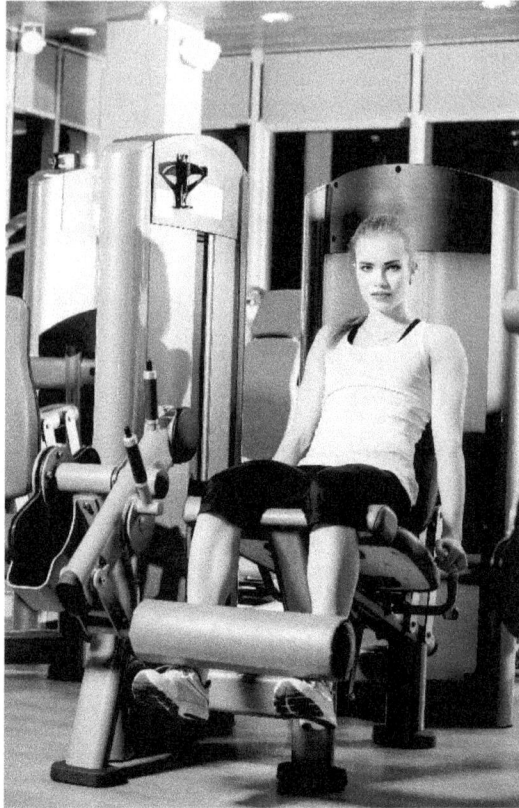

Horizontal leg press machine

Major Muscles worked: Quadriceps/Gluteus Maximus/minimus/Bicep
Femoris/Soleus/Gastrocnemius

- Sit with your back up against the pad, feet shoulder width apart.
- Adjust the seat at or slightly below parallel.
- To increase the emphasis on the hamstrings, place your feet on the upper part on the foot plate.
- To increase the emphasis on calves, place the ball of your feet on the lower portion of the foot plate.

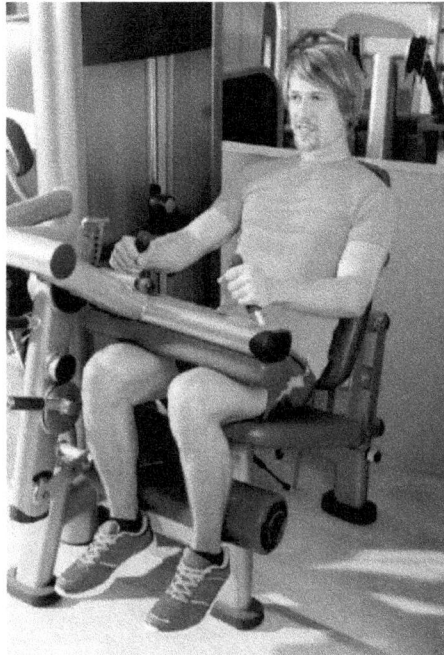

Leg Curl Machine

Major Muscles worked: Bicep Femoris

- Adjust the knee support pad so that your knee is aligned with joint of the machine that connects the lower swing arm to the upper part of the machine.
- Your knee as your leg's pivot point should match the location of the pivot point on the machine.
- Inhale then contract your bicep femoris to perform the exercise.
- Exhale on the downward movement (eccentric).
- Fully extending the ankle downward during this movement mainly works the Bicep Femoris or hamstrings.
- Fully flexing your ankle (foot) up towards your knee during this exercise puts emphasis on your calf muscles

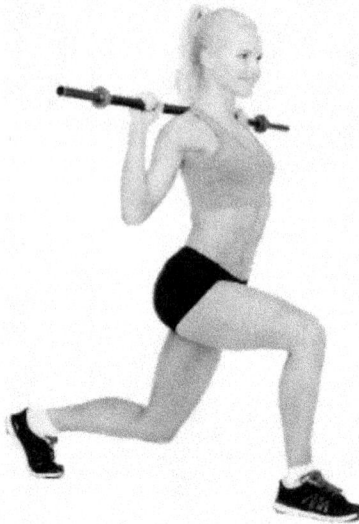

Walking Barbell Lunge

Major Muscles worked: Quadriceps/Gluteus maximus-minimus

- Place the bar on the upper part of your back the same way that you would when performing a squat.
- Keep the upper body upright during the movement.
- Taking a regular step forward, mainly works your quadriceps.
- Taking a longer step forward engages more of your glutes and hamstrings.
- Inhale prior stepping forward.
- Exhale after the movement has been completed.
- Dumbbells or kettlebells can also be used for this movement.

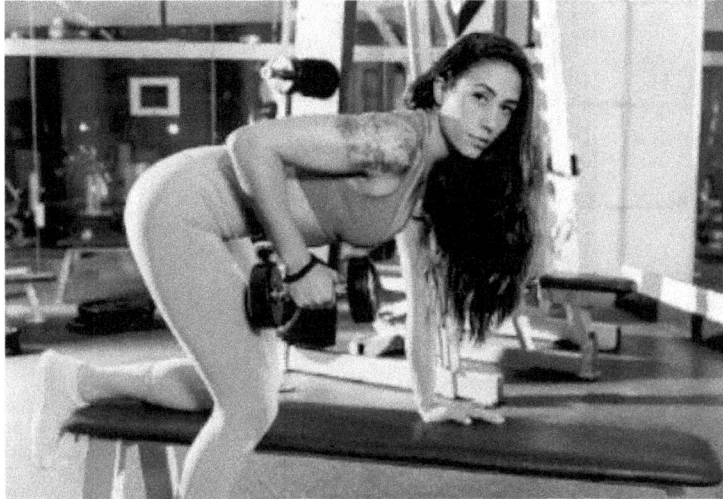

One arm dumbbell row

Major Muscles worked: Latissimus Dorsi/Bicep Femoris

- The foot that is on the same side of your arm that is holding the dumbbell should be planted firmly on the floor.
- Use your opposite arm to support your upper body during the movement.
- Because this a pulling movement, your biceps will also be worked during the movement.
- Inhale prior to the movement.
- Pull the dumbbell up until it is parallel to your waist. Hold for a second and then slowly release the dumbbell to the starting point.
- Exhale when the movement has been completed.
- Repeat for each repetition.

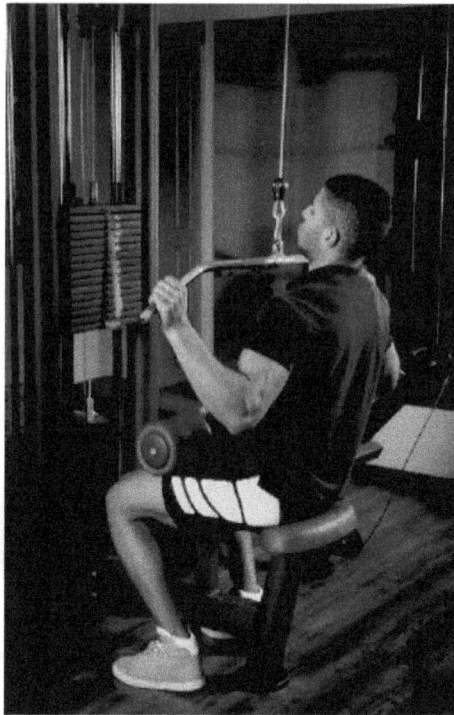

Lateral Pulldown

Major Muscles worked: Latissimus Dorsi/Bicep Femoris

- Grasp the bar with an overhand grip that is slightly wider than shoulder width.
- Keep your body in an upright position; avoid leaning too far forward or backward.
- Pull the bar to just below your chin and just above your upper chest.
- Hold the contraction and slowly let the bar rise back to its starting position.
- Inhale at the start of the movement.
- Exhale at the end of the movement.

Note: I do not suggest attempting to pull the bar behind your head. This may cause impingement. There is also no evidence that pulling the bar behind the head provides greater gains.

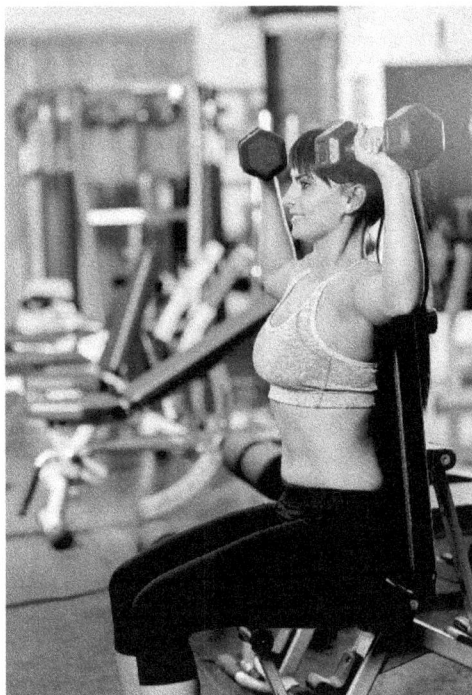

Shoulder Press

Major Muscles worked: Deltoids

- The barbell should be positioned slightly in front and above your head.
- While in a seated position, with palms facing out, grasp the barbell so that your elbows are bent at a 90-degree angle and your hands are shoulder width apart.
- Your back should be straight and your chest forward.
- Inhale, unrack the barbell and slowly lower the barbell to shoulder height.
- Exhale at the end of the movement.
- Ensure that the barbell is not lowered past shoulder height.

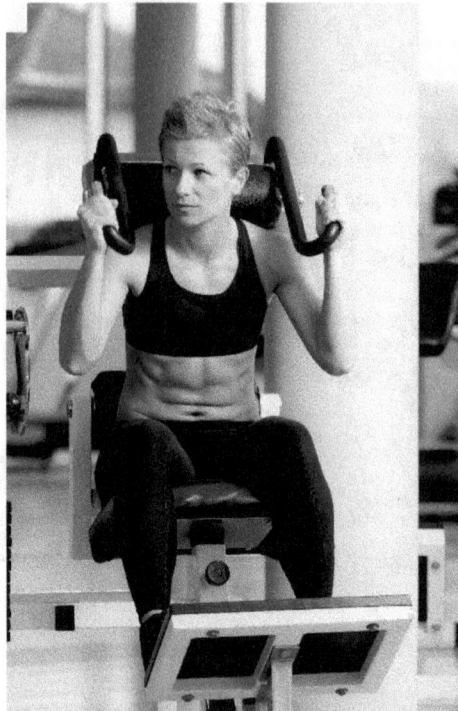

Ab Crunch machine

Muscles worked: Rectus Abdominis

- Adjust the seat height so that the handles are slightly above your shoulders.
- Ensure to round your back during the movement.
- Inhale at the beginning of the movement.
- Exhale while you are contracting your abs.
- Hold the movement in the downward position while holding the contraction for a second.
- Slowly release back to the starting position.

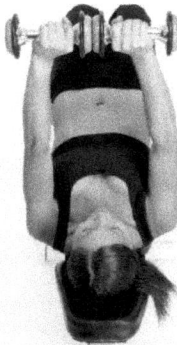

Dumbbell Decline press

Muscles worked: Pectorals/Chest/Triceps brachii

- When laying down on the decline bench, ensure that your feet are properly secured. Some benches have pads that your feet should be secured under. This is your base and helps to produce additional support.
- While still in an upright position, place the dumbbells on top of your legs, palms facing inward. If you have a spotter, your spotter should be able to hand you the dumbbells after you lay down on the bench.
- Slowly lower your upper body down on the bench. You should lay on the blades of your shoulders. There should be a ½ inch to 1-inch space between the bench and your lower back.
- Hold the dumbbells directly above your chest, with your elbows at a 90-degree angle.
- Those with shoulder problems, may find that pressing the dumbbells with your palms facing inward may put less stress on your shoulders. Otherwise, press the dumbbells with your palms facing toward your feet.
- Ensure you keep the dumbbells directly above your chest when you press the dumbbells. If the dumbbells get too far above or below your chest, the pressing movement could put additional stress on your shoulders.
- Exhale on the upward movement (concentric/contraction) and Inhale on the downward movement (eccentric).

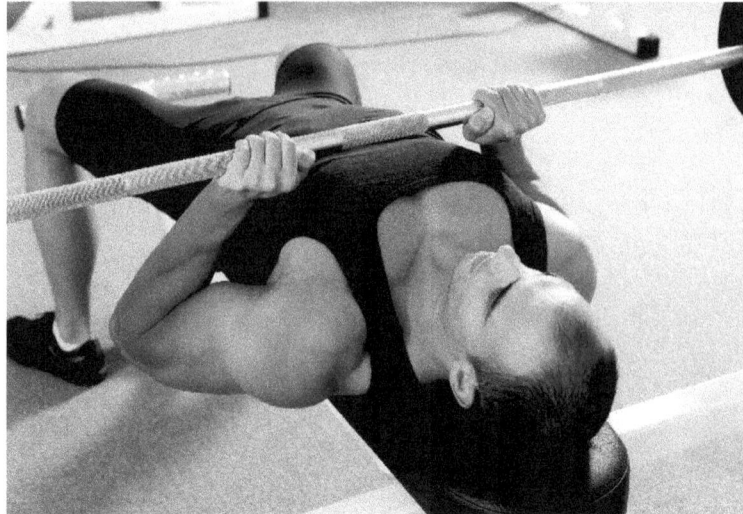

Close grip bench

Muscles worked: Pectorals/Chest/Triceps brachii

- This exercise works the same muscle groups as the bench press does, however, due to the narrower position of the hands, more emphasis is placed on the triceps brachii.
- Keep feet flat on the floor. This is your base and helps to produce additional force.
- Grasp the bar with an overhand grip. The bar should rest just above your wrist, on the heel of your hand. Your hands should be placed on the bar directly above and in between the outer portion of your chest and your shoulders
- You should lay on the blades of your shoulders. There should be a ½ inch to 1-inch space between the bench and your lower back.
- Push the bar, by bringing your elbows closer to your body. Don't by using your shoulders.
- The proper travel of the bar is not in a straight line from your chest, up. The proper travel is actually in a slight curve up towards your head.
- Inhale on the downward movement (eccentric) and exhale on the upward movement (concentric/contraction).
- Avoid performing the Valsava maneuver, which is to hold your breath during the entire movement. When the Valsava maneuver is performed, blood pressure rises significantly which may cause light headedness or dizziness.

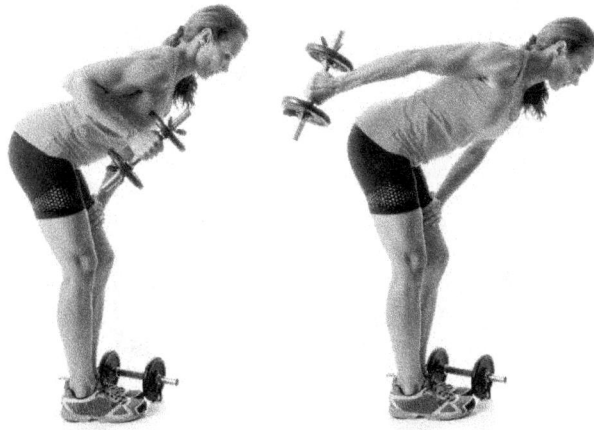

Dumbbell Kickback

Major Muscles worked: Triceps brachii

- You can use a handle or grasp the end of the cable itself. For greater control and maneuverability, I usually grasp the end of the cable instead of using a handle.
- Bend your torso until a 90-degree angle is obtained or your torso is near parallel to the floor.
- The arm that is holding the cable, should also be bent at a 90-degree angle.
- Ensure that your elbow is close your side and not out and away from your body.
- Slowly bend your elbow to the rear, until your arm is fully extended.
- Squeeze your tricep muscle and hold at the end of the movement.
- Slowly release your arm back to the starting position (90-degree angle).

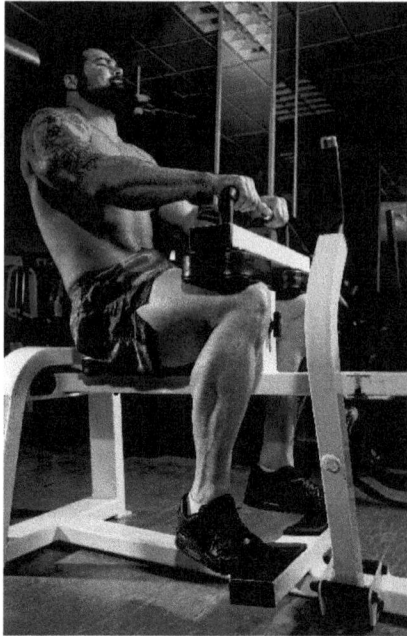

Seated Calf Raise

Muscles worked: Gastrocnemius/Soleus

- Adjust the padding of the machine so that it will allow you to place the lower part of your legs snugly under the padding.
- Sit on the machine and ensure that the locking mechanism is fully functional and in place.
- Slowly unrack the weight.
- Slowly lower the heels of your foot until your calf muscles are fully stretched.
- Ensuring that the balls of your feet are on the platform of the machine, slowly raise your heels until your calf muscles are fully flexed.
- Squeeze your calf muscles at the top of the movement.
- Hold and then repeat the movement.
- You can angle the balls of your feet inward to work more of your outer calves or angle your feet outwards to work your inner calves.

Exercise program for at home or outdoors (using resistance bands)

The same steps that we used for our "in the gym" resistance training program can be used for an at home or outdoor resistance program.

Step 1-Determine the type of resistance training program, based on the principle of specificity. Just as we determined what the focus of the resistance training program for Marilyn would be, the same principle applies when using resistance bands. The resistance training program using resistance bands, that follows, is developed as a 3-day split program.

Step 2-Determine what your 1 repetition maximum is for an exercise that works each major muscle group. Resistance bands can be purchased from weights as little as 2 lbs. to 200 lbs. For simplicity, we'll use the same 1 repetition maximums that we used for Marilyn's free weight program. However, because resistance bands use a free range of motion, unlike selectorized machine, you'll find that the weight that you use for resistance bands might be less. Resistance bands offer some benefits over free weights as well.

Step 3-Again, we'll use the same periodization that we did for the free weight/selectorized machine program. Intensity will be increased every two weeks.

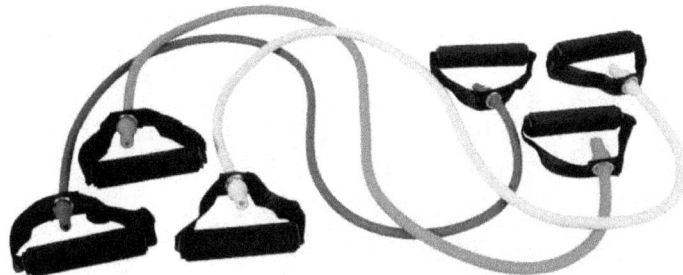

Marilyn's Workout
Week 1-2
Initial Conditioning stage

Day 1	Sets	Intensity	Reps	Day 2	Sets	Intensity	Reps	Day 3	Sets	Intensity	Reps
Warm-up Jog in place/jumping jacks	1	5-6 minutes		Warm-up Jog in place/jumping jacks	1	5-6 minutes		Warm-up Jog in place/jumping jacks	1	5-6 minutes	
Push-up	3	60% or 60lbs	10-12	Front Squat	3	60% or 90lbs	10-12	Lateral pulldown	3	60% or 48lbs	10-12
Standing Chest press	3	60% x 57lbs	10-12	Leg extension	3	60% or 120lbs	10-12	Bent over row	3 x 2	60% or 21lbs	10-12
Narrow-width push-up	3	60% or 66lbs	10-12	Prone leg curl	3	60% or 36lbs	10-12	Overhead press	3	60% or 48lbs	10-12
Tricep kickback	3	60% or 21lbs	10-12	Standing or seated abduction	3	60% or 36lbs	10-12	Lateral raise	3	60% or 21lbs	10-12
Overhead tricep extension	3	60% x 24lbs	10-12	Lunge	3	60% or 42lbs	10-12	Upright row	3 x 2	60% or 12lbs	10-12
Kneeling crunch	3	60% x 48lbs	10-12	Toe raises	3	60% or 72lbs	10-12	Standing bicep curl	3 x 2	60% or 12lbs	10-12
Woodchoppers	3 x 2	60% 18lbs	12-15	Russian twist	3	60% or 60lbs	12-15	Concentration curl	3		12-15
Reverse crunch	3		20-25	Kneeling crunch	3	10lbs ball/dumbbell	15-20	Russian twist	3		15-20
Cool-down		5-6 minutes		Cool-down		5-6 minutes		Cool-down		5-6 minutes	
Stretch				Stretch				Stretch			

138

Marilyn's Workout
Week 3-4
Improvement conditioning phase

Day 1	Sets	Intensity	Reps	Day 2	Sets	Intensity	Reps	Day 3	Sets	Intensity	Reps
Warm-up Jog in place/jumping jacks	1	5-6 minutes		Warm-up Jog in place/jumping jacks	1	5-6 minutes		Warm-up Jog in place/jumping jacks		5-6 minutes	
Push-up	3	70%or 70lbs	10-12	Front Squat	3	70% or 90lbs	10-12	Lateral pulldown	3	70% or 48lbs	10-12
Standing Chest press	3	70%x 57lbs	10-12	Leg extension	3	70% or 120lbs	10-12	Bent over row	3 x 2	70% or 21lbs	10-12
Narrow-width push-up	3	70%or 66lbs	10-12	Prone leg curl	3	70% or 36lbs	10-12	Overhead press	3	70% or 48lbs	10-12
Tricep kickback	3	70%or 21lbs	10-12	Standing or seated abduction	3	70% or 36lbs	10-12	Lateral raise	3	70% or 21lbs	10-12
Overhead tricep extension	3	70%x 24lbs	10-12	Lunge	3	70% or 42lbs	10-12	Upright row	3 x 2	70% or 12lbs	10-12
Kneeling crunch	3	70%x 48lbs	10-12	Toe raises	3	70% or 72lbs	10-12	Standing bicep curl	3 x 2	70% or 12lbs	10-12
Woodchoppers	3 x 2	70%18lbs	12-15	Russian twist	3	70% or 60lbs	12-15	Concentration curl	3		12-15
Reverse crunch	3		20-25	Kneeling crunch	3	10lbs ball/dumbbell	15-20	Russian twist	3		15-20
Cool-down		5-6 minutes		Cool-down		5-6 minutes		Cool-down		5-6 minutes	
Stretch				Stretch				Stretch			

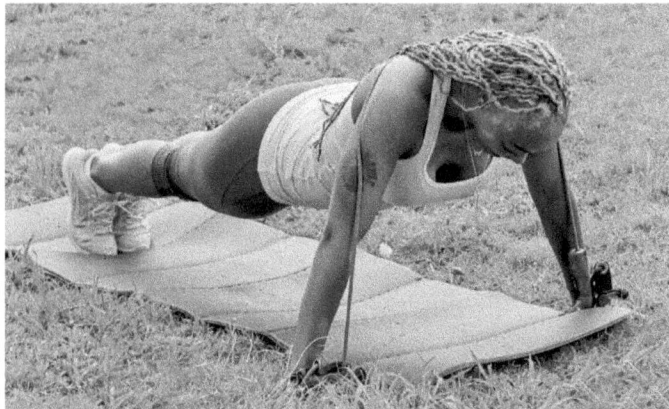

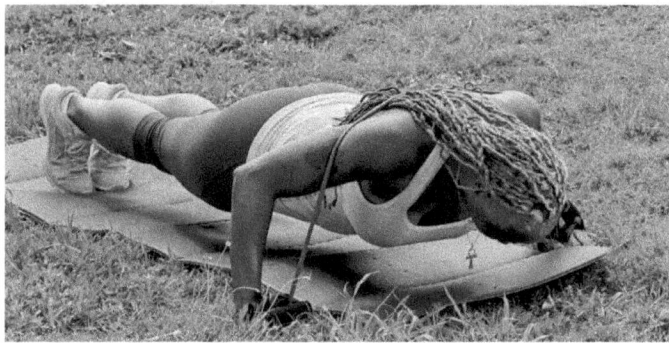

Push-up

Muscles worked: Pectorals/Chest

- Secure the resistance bands by wrapping and then looping the handles around your hands.
- Ensure that the mid-point of the band is securely seated on the upper back (scapula).
- Fully extend your arms to the starting position.
- Slowly lower yourself, while exhaling, during the eccentric movement, until your elbow is slightly less than a 90-degree angle.
- Hold for one second and then slowly push yourself to the starting position, while inhaling. (Concentric).
- Repeat for each repetition.

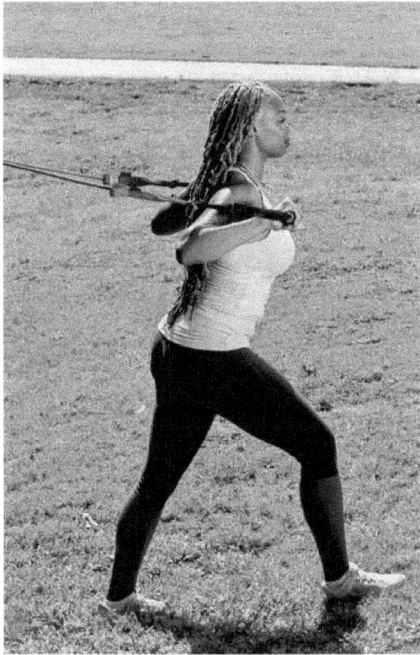

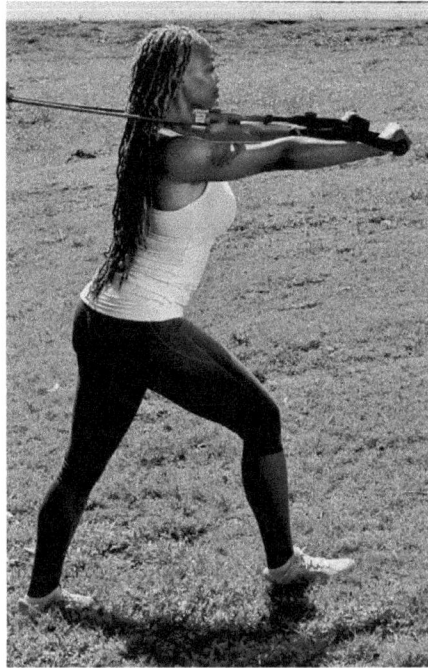

Standing Chest Press

Muscles worked: Pectorals/Chest

- Secure the resistance band by wrapping the band around a tree, pole or other stationary object. Ensure the band is at shoulder height.
- Ensure that your footing is secure. Take one step with either your right or left foot to create your base.
- Start with your hands positioned at shoulder height and slightly in front of your pectoral/chest muscles. Your arms should be parallel to the ground.
- Fully extend your arms while keeping them parallel to the ground. Exhale during the concentric movement. Hold for one second.
- Slowly bring your hands and arms back to the starting position, while inhaling on the eccentric movement.
- Repeat for each repetition.

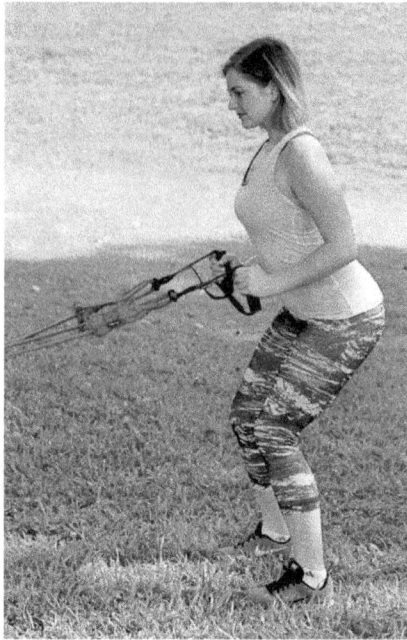

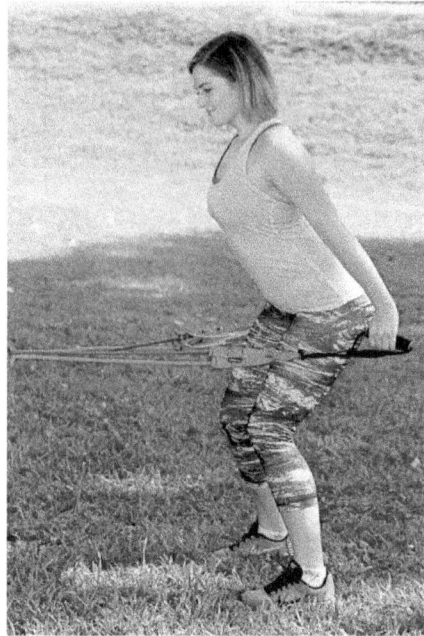

Tricep Kickback

Major Muscles worked: Triceps brachii. All three heads of the tricep muscle group.

- Secure the resistance band by wrapping the band around a tree, pole or other stationary object.
- Ensure the resistance band is at waist height.
- Bend slightly at the knees to create your base. Your feet should be shoulder width apart.
- Hold your arms at a 90-degree angle with your palms facing toward each other.
- Inhale and then fully bend your arms at the elbow creating a 180-degree angle. During this concentric movement, your hands should slightly rotate until your palms are facing behind you. Hold for one second.
- Exhale while you slowly return your hands and arms to the starting position.
- Repeat for each repetition.

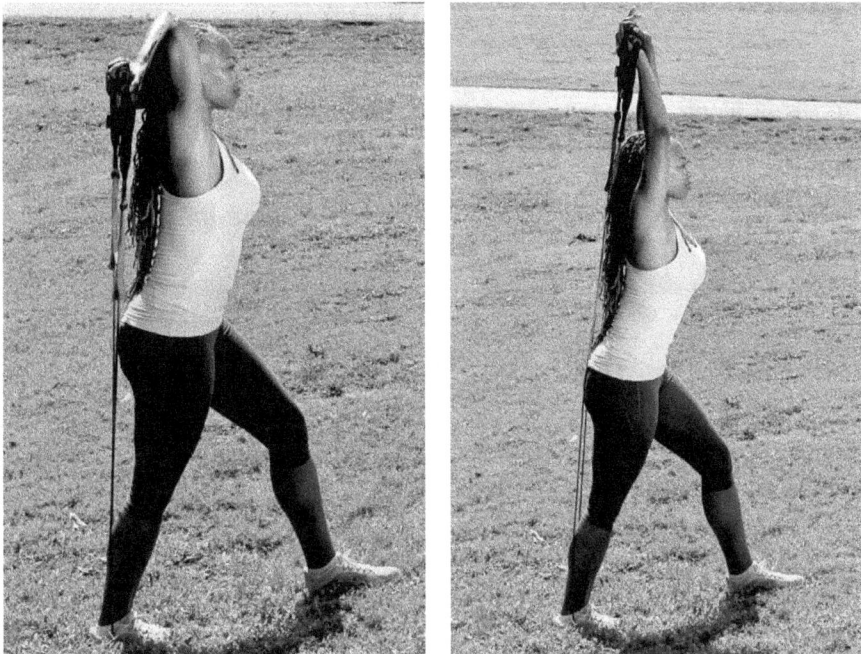

Overhead Tricep extension

Muscles worked: Triceps brachii. All three heads of the tricep muscle group.

- Secure the resistance band by wrapping and looping the band around your back foot.
- Create your base by placing your right or left foot forward. Your bodyweight should be evenly distributed on both feet.
- Hold the resistance band handles at the height of your scapula and/or trapezius. Your arms should be at an approximate angle of 10 degrees and bent only at the elbow.
- Exhale and then fully extend your arms at the elbow creating a 180-degree angle. Hold for one second.
- Slowly decrease the angle by returning your hands and arms to the starting position. Do not allow the resistance band to pull your hands and arms to the starting position at a fast rate. Control the movement. Inhale during this eccentric movement.
- Repeat for each repetition.

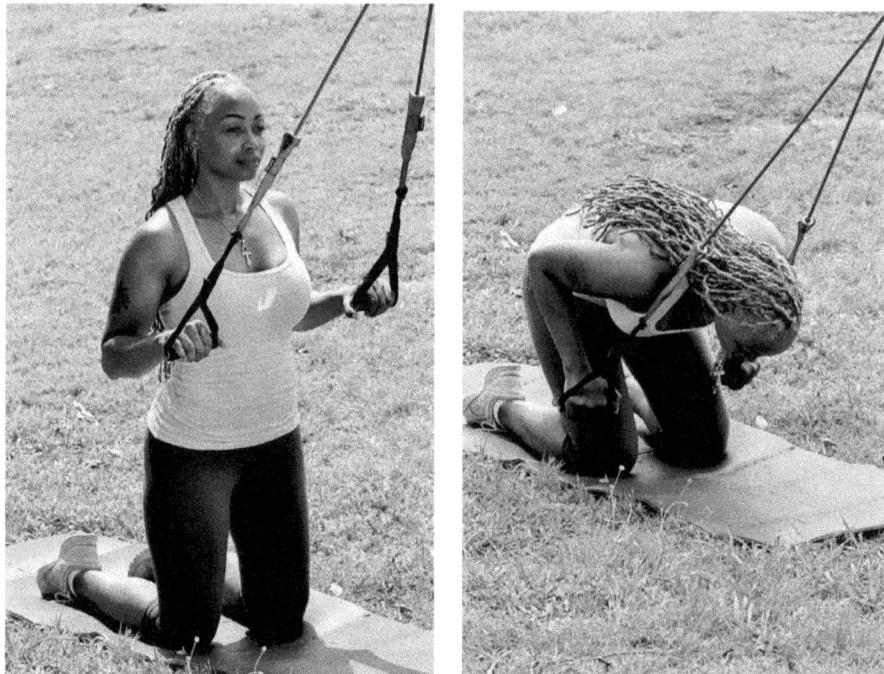

Kneeling Crunch

Muscles worked: Rectus Abdominis

- Secure the resistance band by wrapping the band around a tree, pole or other stationary object. The resistance band should be secured at a height that is above your head.
- Kneel down and secure the handles of the resistance bands by bending your elbows at a 90-degree angle. Your palms should be facing down.
- Bend at your waist and exhale during the concentric movement. Keep your elbows bent at a 90-degree angle. Hold for one second.
- Slowly return to the starting position. Inhale during the eccentric movement.
- Repeat for each repetition.

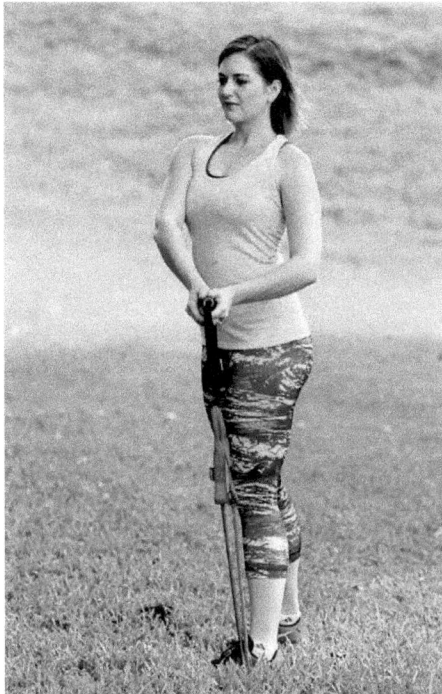

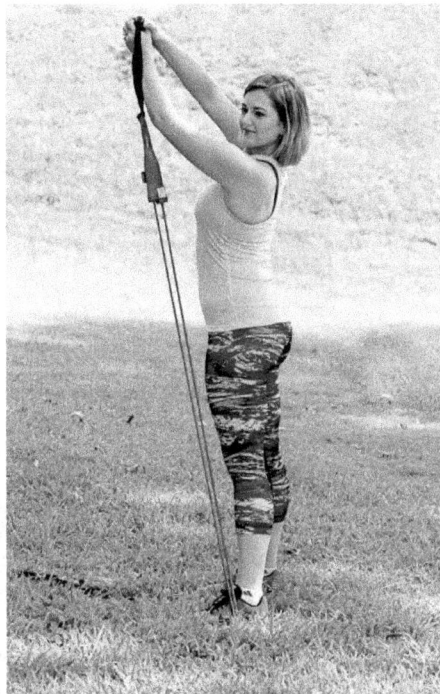

Woodchopper

Muscles worked: Rectus Abdominus/Obliques

- Secure the resistance band by wrapping and looping the band around the foot which is closest to the side that you will be starting with or the side that is opposite to the side that you will be rotating to.

- Hold the handle(s) of the resistance band at waist height. Ensure that the slack has been removed from the band. In order to remove the slack in the band, you may have to wrap or loop more of the resistance band around and/or under your foot.

- In one motion, slowly raise your arms and hands above your head and twist your torso to the opposite side. Exhale during this movement. Hold for one second.

- Inhale and slowly return to the starting position.
- Repeat for each repetition. Switch sides.

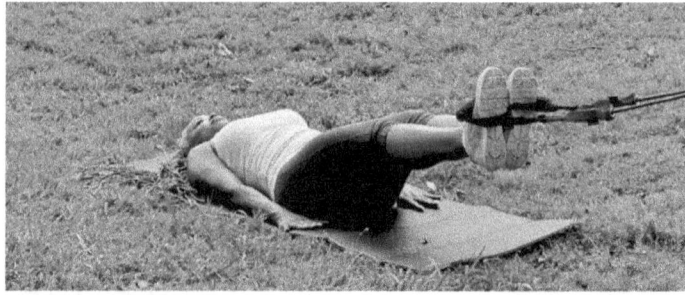

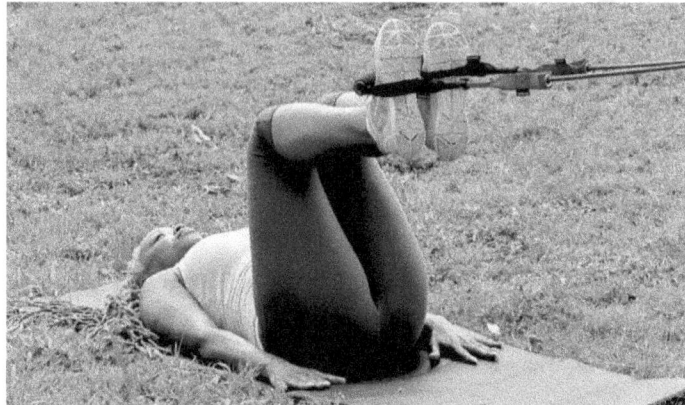

Reverse Crunch

Muscles worked: Rectus Abdominis

- Secure the resistance band by wrapping one end of the band around a tree, pole or other stationary object.
- Secure the other end of the resistance band by wrapping or looping the handles around your feet.
- Lay on your back (supine position) with your legs raised at or near a 45-degree angle.
- While inhaling, pull your knees toward your chest while squeezing your abdomen. Stop the movement when your upper leg is at a 90-degree angle. Hold the movement for one second.
- While exhaling, return your legs to the starting position.
- Repeat for each repetition

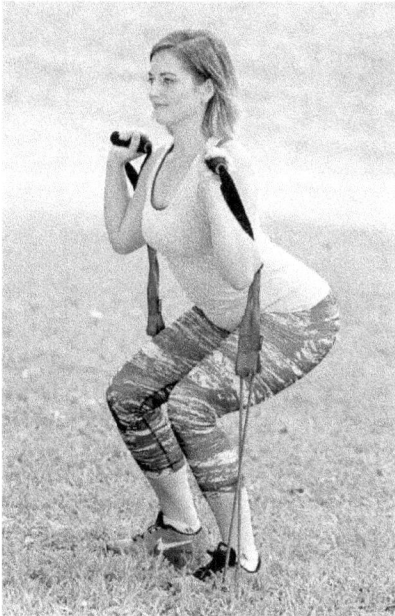

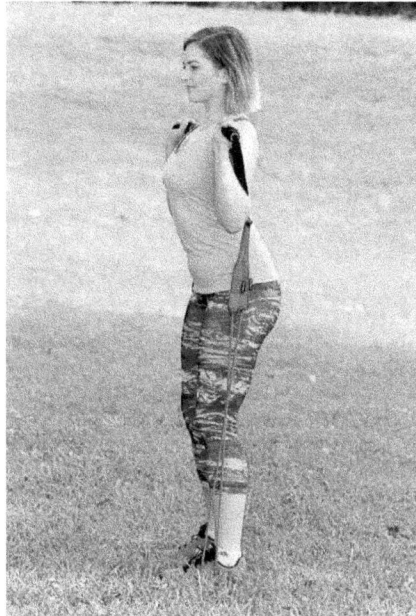

Front Squat
Muscles worked: Quadriceps/Gluteus Maximus-minimus/Bicep Femoris

- Secure the resistance band by placing the midpoint of the band under the midpoint of your foot.
- Hold the band at shoulder height. You can use your arms (elbows) to help to keep the band stationary.
- It is best to start this exercise from a squatting position, so that you can ensure that all of the slack has been taken out of the band.
- While exhaling, stand up while holding the resistance band in place. Hold the movement for one second.
- While inhaling, return to the starting position.
- Repeat for each repetition

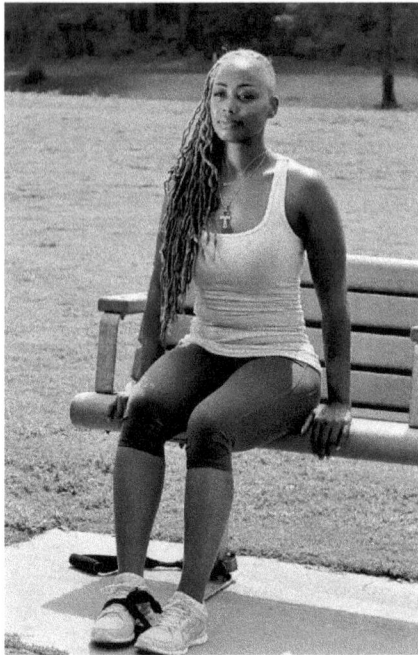

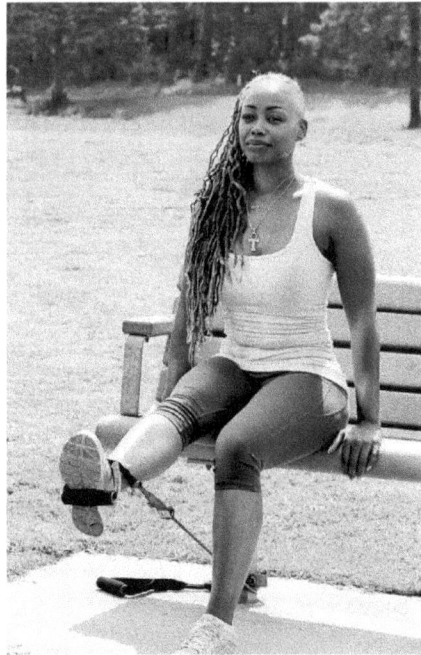

Leg Extension

Muscles worked: Quadriceps

- Secure one end of the resistance band around the leg of a park bench or other stationary object.
- Secure the other end of the resistance band by wrapping/looping the handle of the band around your foot.
- Sit with your back erect and your legs at a 90-degree angle. You may hold onto the edge of the bench for added support.
- While exhaling, bend your leg at the knee, creating a 180-degree angle. Hold for one second.
- While inhaling, return your leg to the starting position.
- Repeat for each repetition. Switch legs.

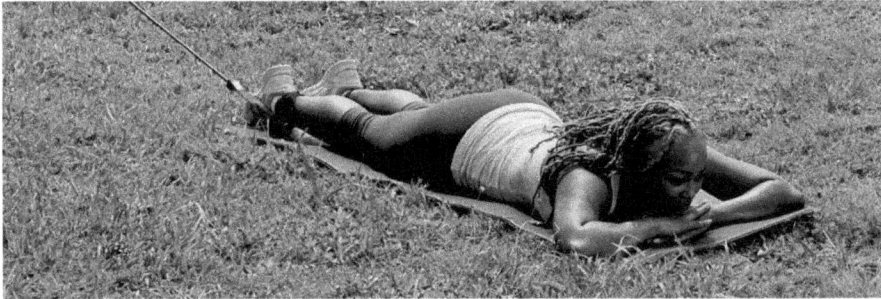

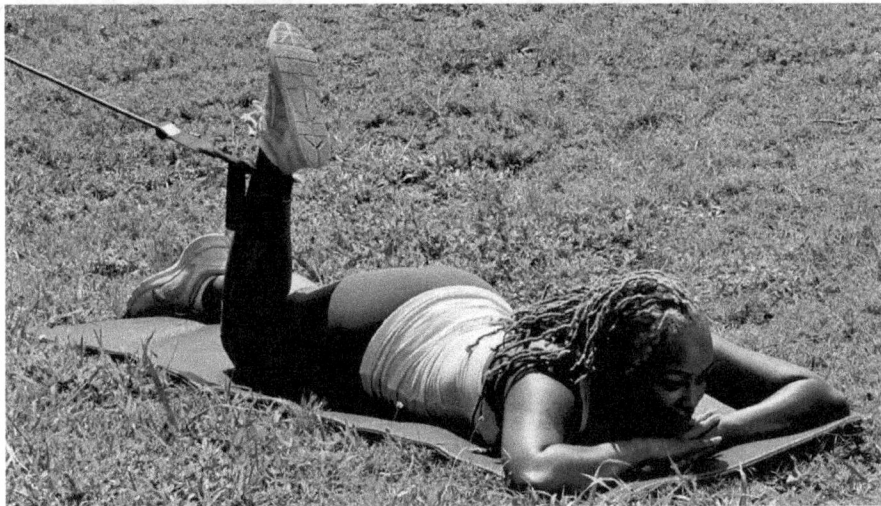

Prone Leg Curl

Muscles worked: Bicep Femoris

- Secure the resistance band by wrapping one end of the band around a tree, pole or other stationary object.
- Lay down on your stomach (prone position)
- Secure the other end of the resistance band by wrapping/looping the handle of the band around your foot.
- While exhaling, curl your leg to form a 90-degree angle. Hold for one second.
- While inhaling, slowly lower your leg to the starting position.
- Repeat for each repetition. Switch legs.

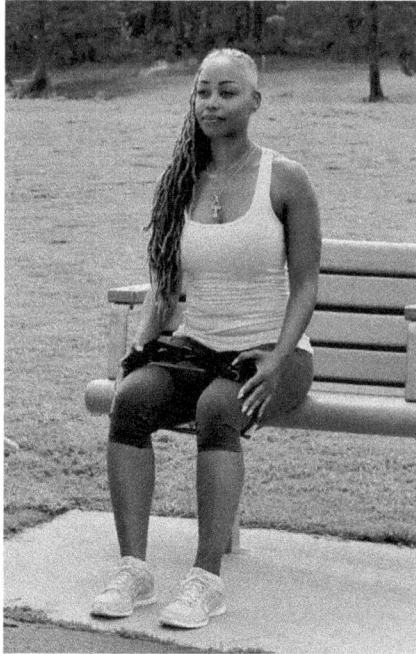

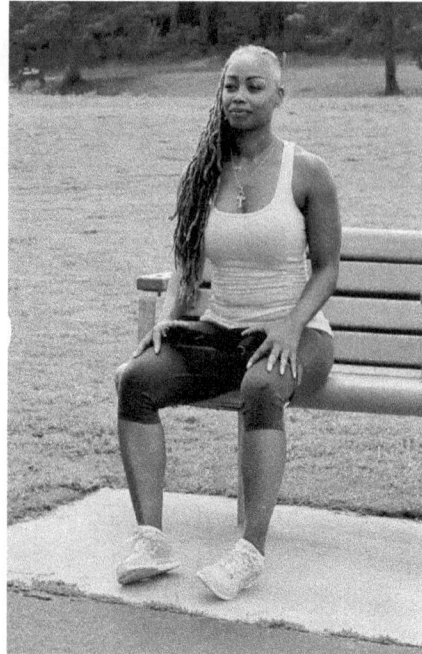

Sitting Abductor
Muscles worked: Glutes Maximus/Minimus-Rectus Femoris

- Secure the resistance band by wrapping the band around the middle of your upper legs. The distance between your right and left leg should be no more than 2-3 inches.
  Ensure that all of the slack is taken out of the resistance band.
- While exhaling, slowly push your legs/thighs outward, to as far as you can. You can roll your feet outward to assist you with this movement. Hold for one second.
- While inhaling, slowly release your legs/thighs to the starting position.
- Repeat for each repetition.

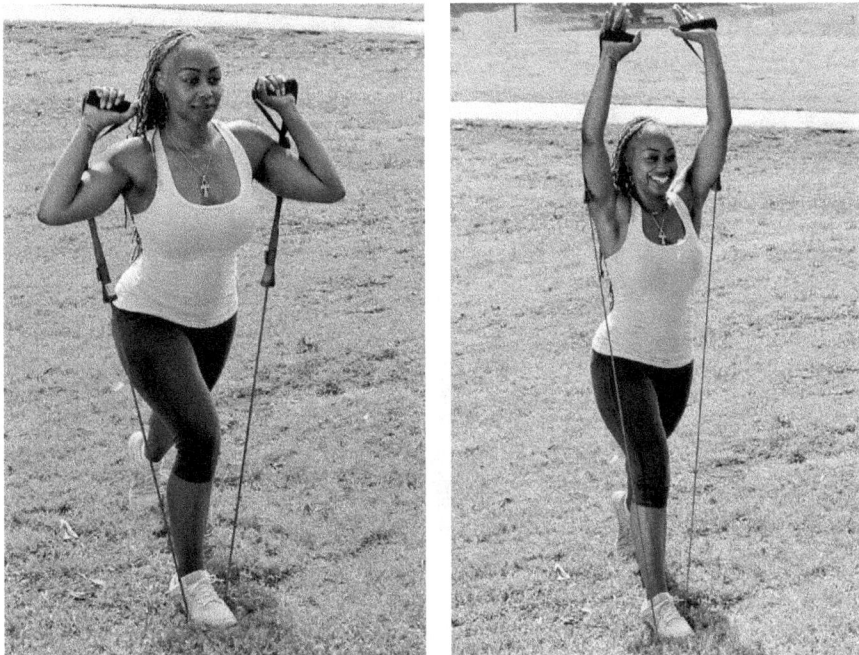

Lunge
Muscles worked: Quadriceps/Rectus Femoris/ Gluteus Maximus/Minimus

- Stand with one leg six to eight inches in front of you and one leg six to eight inches behind you. This is your base. Your bodyweight should be evenly distributed on both feet.
- Secure the resistance band by wrapping/looping the midpoint of the band around your front foot.
- Hold the resistance band at shoulder height.
- While exhaling, in one smooth and controlled motion, squat down toward your foot that is in front of you and push the resistance band up.
- While inhaling, slowly return to the starting position.
- Repeat for each repetition. Switch sides.

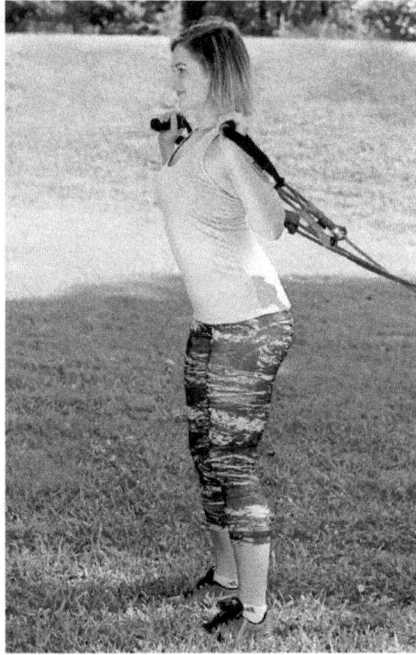

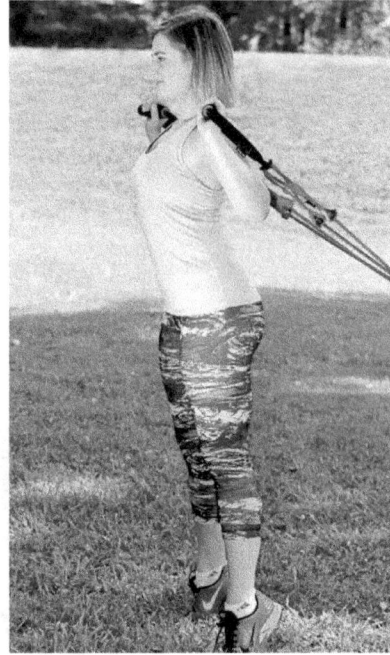

Toe (Heel) raise

Muscles worked: Gastrocnemius/Soleus

- Secure the resistance band by wrapping one end of the band around a tree, pole or other stationary object. Ensure that the slack is taken out of the band by moving further away from the band.
- Hold the resistance band at shoulder height.
- While exhaling, lift the heels of your foot until you are standing on the balls of your feet. Hold for one second.
- While inhaling, slowly return to the starting position.
- Repeat for each repetition.

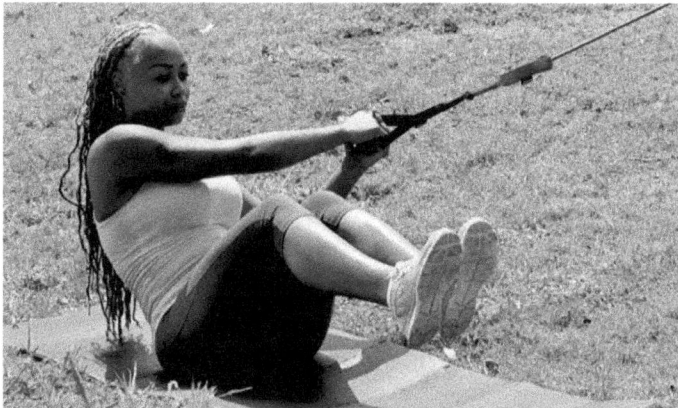
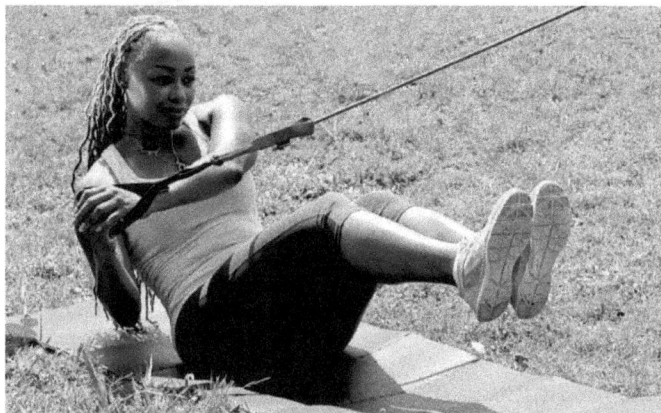

Russian Twist
Muscles worked: Obliques/Rectus Abdominis

- Secure the resistance band by wrapping one end of the band around a tree, pole or other stationary object.
- While in a seated position, raise your legs to a 30-degree angle. Hold the resistance band on the same side of where the band is secured.
- While exhaling, rotate your torso to the opposite side of where the band is secured. Hold for one second.
- While inhaling, return to the starting position.
- Repeat for each repetition. Switch sides.

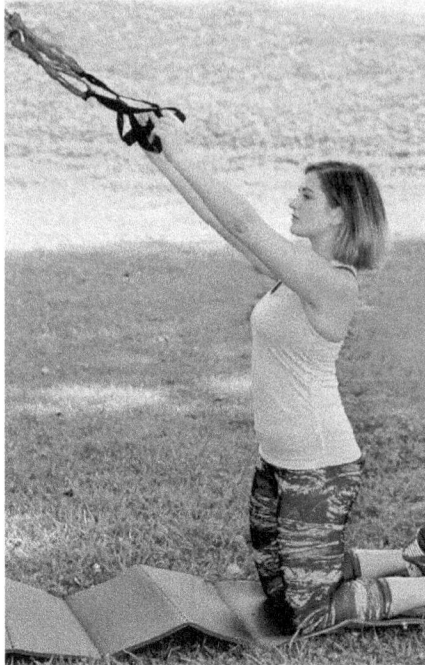

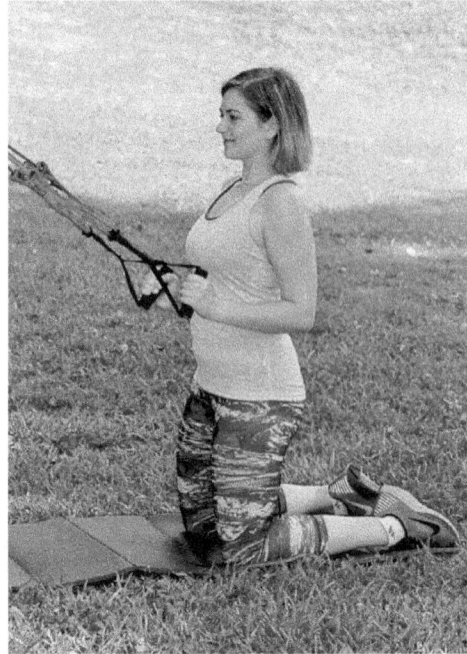

Lateral Pulldown

Muscles worked: Latissimus Dorsi

- Secure the resistance band by wrapping one end of the band around a tree, pole or other stationary object.
- While in a kneeling position, hold the resistance band at a 30-degree angle, out front and above your head.
- While exhaling, pull the resistance bands down to your abdomen, until your arms are at a 90-degree angle. Hold for one second.
- While inhaling, slowly return to the starting position.
- Repeat for each repetition.

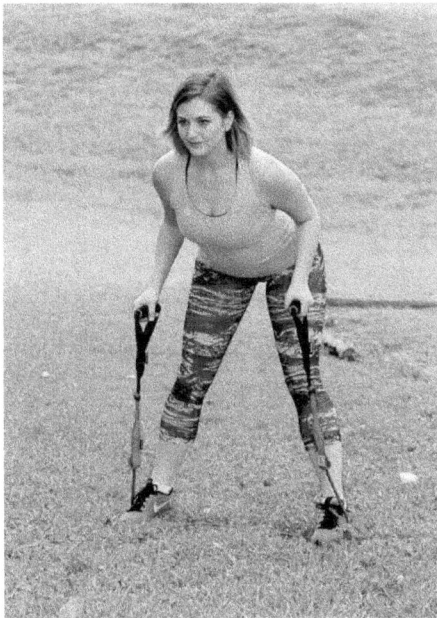

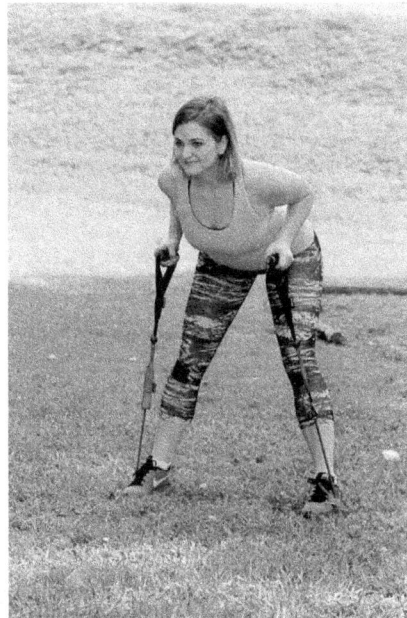

Bent over row

Muscles worked: Latissimus Dorsi

- Secure the resistance band by placing the midpoint of the band under the midpoint of both of your feet.
- Your feet should be slightly wider than shoulder width apart. To decrease the slack in the resistance band, you may need to widen your stance.
- Lean your torso forward until you reach a 90-degree angle.
- Hold the handles of the resistance band at or slightly below knee height.
- While exhaling, pull the resistance band up to your abdomen. Hold for one second.
- While inhaling, slowly return to the starting position.
- Repeat for each repetition.

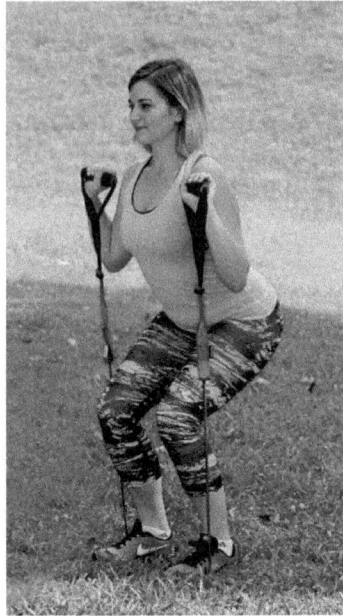

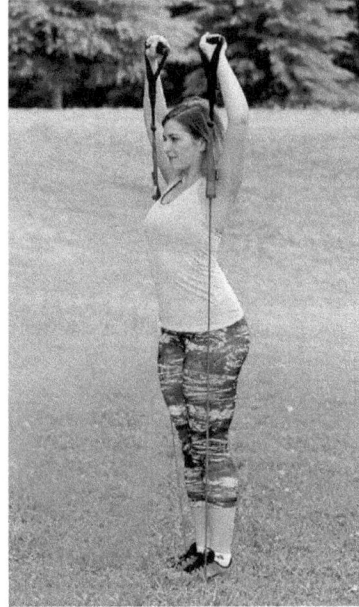

Overhead press

Muscles worked: Deltoids

- Secure the resistance band by placing the midpoint of the band under the midpoint of both of your feet.
- Your feet should be shoulder width apart.
- You will actually start this movement in a squatted position.
- Hold the resistance band at shoulder height.
- While exhaling and in one motion, stand and push the resistance band up, above your head. Hold for one second.
- While inhaling, slowly return to the starting position.
- Repeat for each repetition

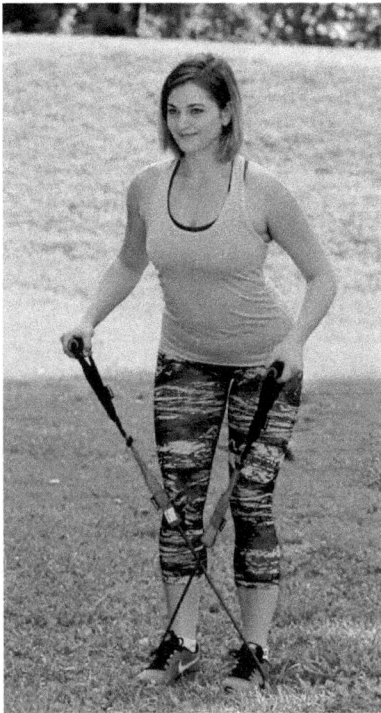

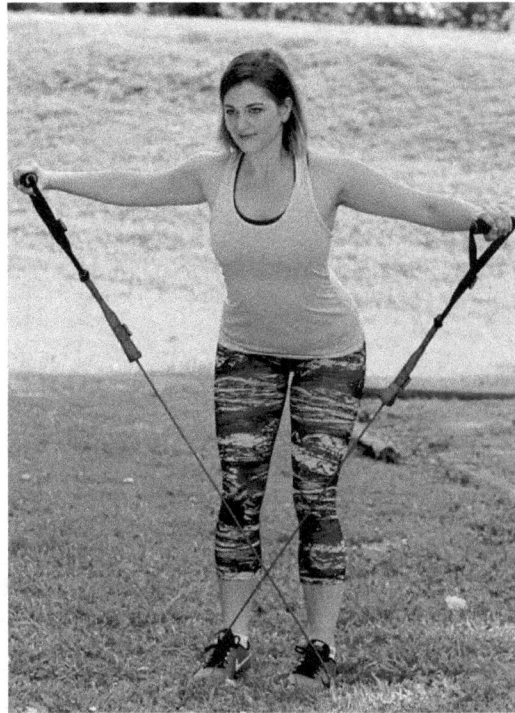

Lateral Raise

Muscles worked: Deltoids (medial)

- Secure the resistance band by placing the midpoint of the band under the midpoint of both of your feet.
- Make an X with the cross by placing the right handle in your left hand and the left handle in your right hand.
- Lean your torso slightly forward until you reach a 10-15-degree angle.
- While exhaling, slowly raise the handles of the resistance band until your arms create a 180-degree angle (or are at the same height as your shoulders). Hold for one second.
- While inhaling, slowly lower your arms until you reach the starting position.
- Repeat for each repetition

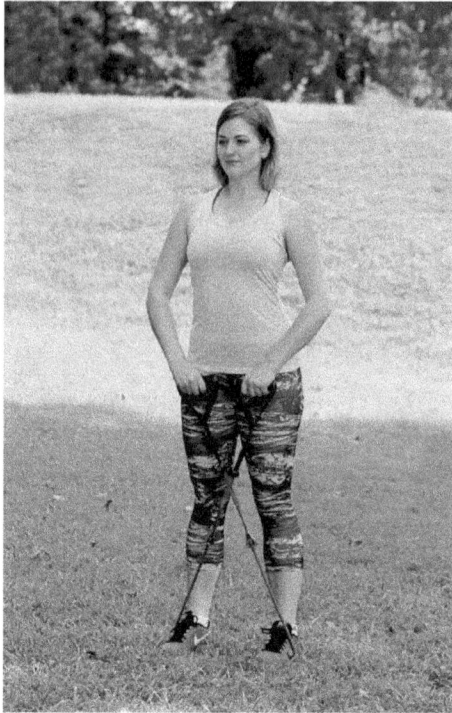

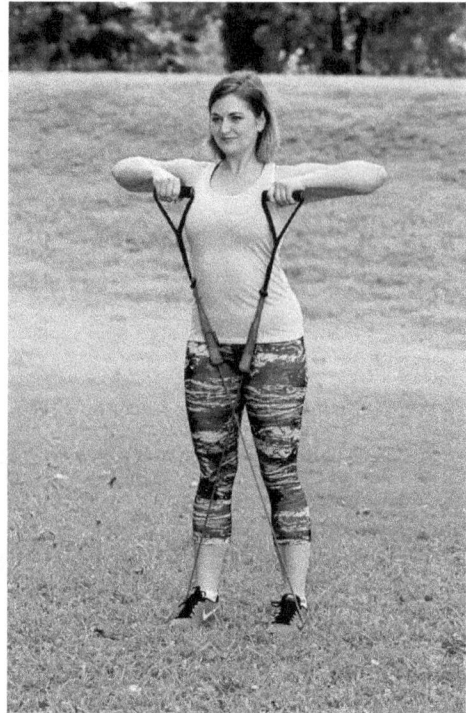

Upright row

Muscles worked: Deltoids (Anterior)

- Secure the resistance band by placing the midpoint of the band under the midpoint of both of your feet.
- Make an X with the cross by placing the right handle in your left hand and the left handle in your right hand.
- Hold the resistance band at waist height.
- While exhaling, pull the resistance band up to shoulder height. Hold for one second.
- While inhaling, slowly return to the starting position.
- Repeat for each repetition.

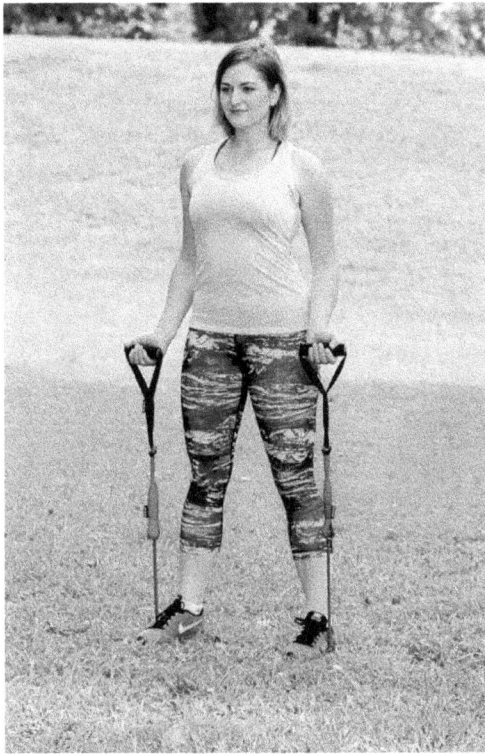

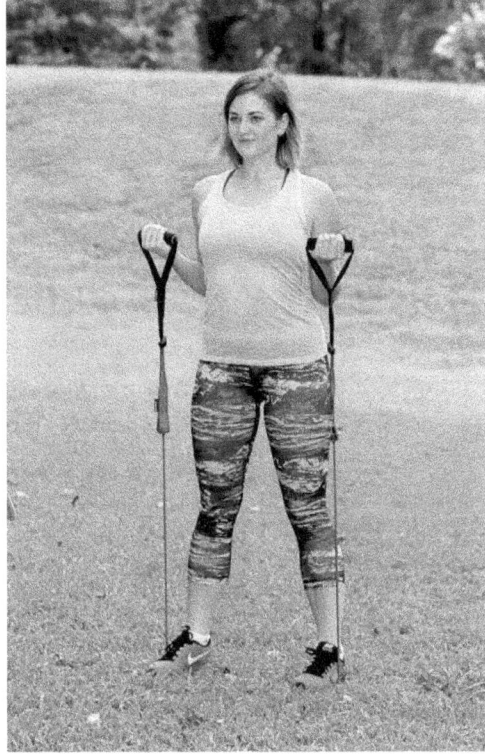

Bicep curl

Muscles worked: Bicep brachii

- Secure the resistance band by placing the midpoint of the band under the midpoint of both of your feet.
- Hold the resistance band at waist height with your palms facing outward.
- While exhaling, bend your elbows until your arms reach a 15-20-degree angle. Hold for one second.
- While inhaling, slowly return to the starting position.
- Repeat for each repetition.

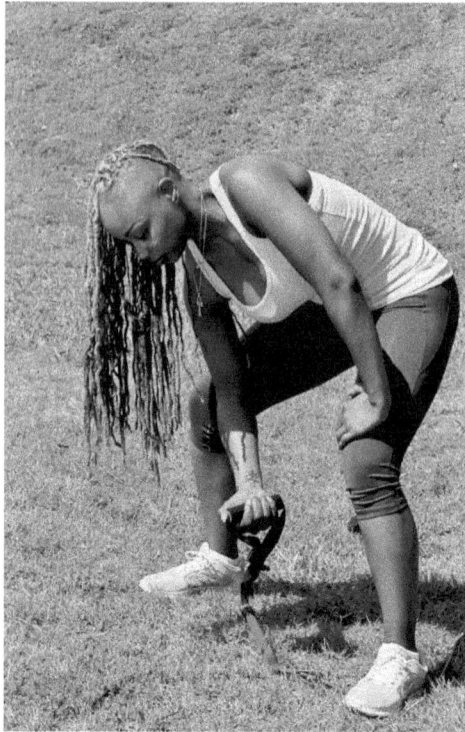

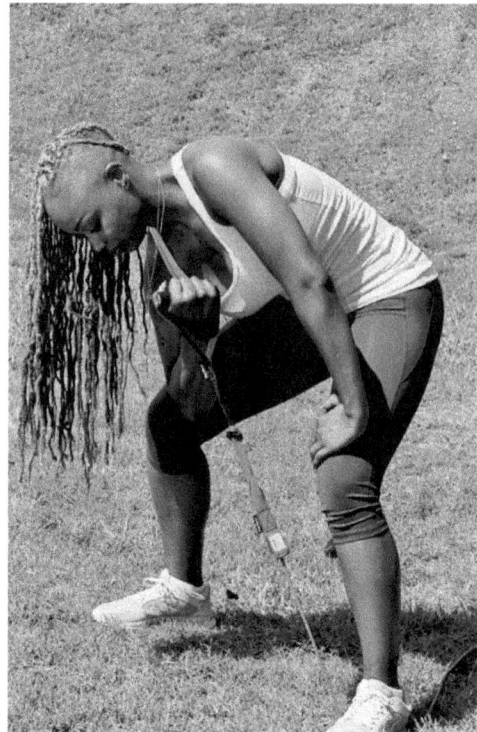

Concentration Curl

Muscles worked: Bicep brachii

- Secure the resistance band by placing most of the band under your left foot, while ensuring that you take the slack out of the band.
- Lean your torso forward and place your left hand on your leg (right above your knee) for added support.
- While exhaling, slowly bend your elbow until your arm reaches a 10-15-degree angle. Your palm should be facing inward during this movement. Hold for one second.
1. While inhaling, slowly return to the starting position.
- Repeat for each repetition. Switch sides.

Chapter 5

Myth Busters

Live,

    Learn,

        Imagine,

            Achieve.

               George Dorsey

This chapter is dedicated to dispelling some of the many myths that are spread throughout the health and fitness industry.

1. I don't want to lift heavy weights because I don't want to look like a man.

Unfortunately, many women shy away from incorporating a resistance training program into their workout regimen. Most women would prefer to take group aerobic type classes than spend any time around free weights. And this is where it all goes wrong. For starters, the body of a woman can't generate the same amount of testosterone that the body of a male can. The ovaries of a woman produce both testosterone and estrogen. Testosterone is a hormone that can control sex drive, regulate sperm production, promote muscle mass, increase energy and can influence behavior. The chart below shows the differences in testosterone levels between men and women. Second, research has proven that women have a higher prevalence of sarcopenia (age induced muscle wasting) and osteoporosis than men.18 A resistance training program along with the proper nutrition program and help to minimize the effects of both of these diseases in women. Women…. I'll see you in the weight room.

Conclusion: Myth

Age[61]	Female T level (ng/dl):	Male T level (ng/dl):
0-5 months	20-80	75-400
6 mos.-9 yrs	<7-20	<7-20
10-11 yrs.	<7-44	<7-130
12-13 yrs		<7-800
12-16 yrs	<7-75	
14 yrs.		<7-1,200
17-18yrs	20-75	
17-18 yrs		300-1,200
19+ yrs	8-60	240-950
Average adult	15-70	270-1,070

2. **I can't eat after 6 pm or I'll gain weight.** Remember the earlier discussion on the first rule of thermodynamics? Any excess energy (calories) will be stored, regardless of when it's consumed. For example, if you've calculated your TDEE to be 2,000 calories and you've already consumed 2,000 calories by 6 pm but you eat another 500 calorie meal, you'll more than likely start to gain weight. If it's 6 pm and you've only eaten 1,500 calories, then another 500 calories will fit nicely into your 2,000 calorie TDEE.

Even when you are sleeping your body is still metabolizing substrates. If you're in a building phase, it's good to have something in your stomach to prevent your body from catabolizing itself. You should focus more on what you eat, rather than what time you eat it. Healthy foods are always best, no matter what time of day it is.

Conclusion: Myth

3. **To get abs to show, I need to do hundreds of crunches.** It doesn't matter how many crunches, Russian twist or leg raises that you do, your body fat has to be within the right body fat percentage in order to see the muscles beneath your skin. Men need to get their body fat percent between 7% to 9% and women 13% to 15%. Men with body fat percentages in the upper ranges find it harder to reach these lower level percentages because men mostly gain their body fat in their abdomen. So what can you do?

- **Increase your cardio!** In order to burn body fat, you have to move. The American College of Sports Medicine (ACSM) recommends that you partake in an aerobic activity 3-4 days per week at 30%-80% of VO2R or Heart Rate Reserve for at least 20-90 minutes.

- **Increase your protein intake.** For information on what type and how much protein to consume, see our post, "Protein: The building block for muscles".

- **Develop a resistance training.** ACSM recommends that you perform resistance training at least 2-3 days per week with 8-10 exercises consisting of 1-4 sets and 8-12 repetitions for each exercise. Your resistance training program should also be developed based on the principles of specificity, overload and reversibility. In short, specificity means that you train for a specific purpose. Overload means that you need to continually attempt to overload the muscle/muscle group. Reversibility means that if you don't use it, you'll lose it.

Conclusion: Myth

4. **I shouldn't eat any carbohydrates, while I am trying to lose weight.** As discussed in earlier in this book, carbohydrates are an essential macronutrient that the body uses for a variety of functions. The most important use for carbohydrates is to fuel brain

activity. There are some who think that the human body, to include the brain, can create energy from the metabolism of body fat. Unfortunately, this couldn't be further from the truth. What is most important to know is that your brain is responsible for controlling every bodily function to include reflexes, movement, vision, hearing, and cognitive and mental abilities. The brain is a super user of energy and uses almost 25% of the glucose that is circulating through our body. That's a large consumption of energy considering that the brain is only 3% of our body weight.[35]

Some have used a process called Ketosis to burn body fat while virtually eliminating consumption of carbohydrates. Ketosis occurs when your body is depleted of glucose and uses body fat instead of glucose for energy. The byproduct of this process is called ketones. Unfortunately, ketosis can be dangerous and may cause a disease called ketoacidosis. Ketoacidosis occurs when there is a high accumulation of ketones in the blood. Ketoacidosis can cause dehydration, poor appetite and even loss of consciousness.[62] Research has shown that eating carbohydrates with a low glycemic index number prior to exercising increases fat oxidation as compared to eating foods that have a high glycemic index number.

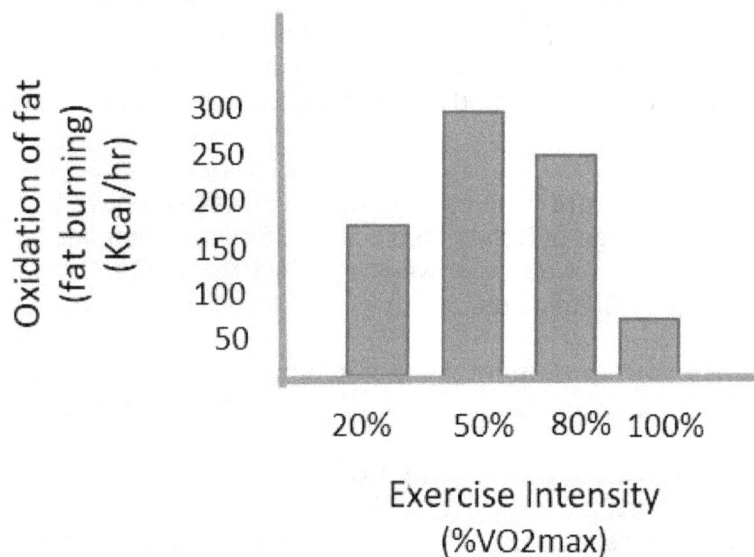

As the chart above shows, body fat can be burned at a higher rate when exercise intensities are above 50% of VO2max. [32]

As you can see consuming the proper amount of carbohydrates is key to achieving good health. So eat those carbs!!!!
Conclusion: Myth

5. **I need to feel pain in order for me to improve my fitness and performance levels.**

How many times have we heard the saying, "No pain, no gain"? There are quite a few people who believe that if they don't feel a significant amount of pain during or after their workouts, then the workouts weren't successful.

There are at three types of pain or exercise-induced muscle damage (EIMD) that you may feel as a result of exercise, acute, DOMS, and chronic.[63] Acute pain occurs during the workout. If you feel pain while exercising, then you should stop your workout immediately to prevent injury. You should then determine the cause of the acute pain. Acute pain can be felt while over exerting a muscle, ligament or tendon. Acute pain can also be caused by pushing a joint past its normal range of motion.

DOMS or delayed onset muscle soreness, may occur 12 to 72 hours after working out. According to ACSM, DOMS may be caused by microscopic damage to muscle fibers that were being worked during the exercise. ACSM also states that DOMS appears to be a side effect of the repair process which occurs as a result of the damage to the muscle fibers.[64]

There are a number of methods that can be used to help reduce the level of pain that is felt after exercising.

- Use of compression garments-A study published in the journal Medicine and Science in Sports and Exercise found that trained men experienced significantly faster recovery. Faster recovery equals a shorter duration of pain that might be felt after exercising.

- Fish oil-A study published in the Clinical Journal of Sport Medicine found that fish oil which included omega-3 fatty acids reduced DOMS in the 48 hours after exercising.

- Use of a non-steroidal anti-inflammatory-In a study conducted by the Department of Health Sciences at Lehman College and published in the Journal of Sports Medicine, periodic use of a nonsteroidal anti-inflammatory drug states that these types of drugs are routinely prescribed to treat EIMD. [65]

- Kinesiology tape-Fairly new on the scene, kinesiology tape or "K-tape" is said to lift skin away from soft tissue to promote greater blood flow to minor injuries for faster recovery. A study in the Journal of Physiotherapy found that study participants who used the k-tape to nonspecific lumbar back pain experienced greater improvement in disability, better trunk endurance and decreased pain compared to those who did not use the k-tape.

- Contrast shower-As a former football player, I'm very familiar with using cold therapy (ice tub) to help to reduce inflammation that may occur after a full day of two-a-days practice. Using a contrast shower works in a similar way. By alternating between hot and cold water (3:1 duration ratio) causes your body to push metabolic waste out of cells and reduce inflammation. A study in the Journal of Strength and Conditioning Research found that this method helped subjects to regain full muscle function after a strenuous workout.

- Epsom salt bath-A Epsom salt bath is probably one of the most widely known home remedies for reducing pain and inflammation after performing strenuous exercise. Research has shown for just a few dollars, an Epsom salt bath can reduce inflammation, regulate electrolytes and improve nerve, muscle and enzyme functioning.

- Stop exercising-The quickest way to reduce any type of pain is to simply stop exercising. However, it is normal to feel some pain after exercising so don't let a little pain discourage your from reaching your goals.

- Reduce the weight-Pain might be caused because too much weight is being used. Reducing the weight that is being used in an exercise to a more manageable weight can help to reduce both and injury.

- Seek medical treatment-If the pain that is felt during a workout or after workout is too much to bear, then certainly seek medical attention.

Feeling some slight pain after a workout is a part of the normal process that your body goes through for growth. However, too much pain can be an indicator of overexertion or injury.

Conclusion: Myth (Partially)

6. **I only need a few hours a sleep a night in order to be healthy.**

The Center of Disease Control estimates that there are 50-70 million adults in America who have a sleep or wakefulness disorder. The number of hours that we sleep dropped by 2.2 hours from 9 hours a century ago to 6.8 hours. The fast paced economy and seemingly endless task list continues to consume more and more of our time, making it harder for your bodies to maintain metabolic and hormonal equilibrium. Sleep disorders can range include:

- Night Terrors
- Obstructive Sleep Apnea
- Central Sleep Apnea
- Insomnia
- Parasomnia
- Narcolepsy

- Teeth Grinding (Bruxism)
- circadian Rhythm Sleep Disorder
- Sleep Paralysis
- Sleep-related eating disorders
- Shift Work Sleep disorders

Studies have shown that sleep deprivation can affect glucose metabolism and hormones such as leptin and ghrelin. Sleep deprivation has shown to decrease leptin, which is a hormone that decreases appetite and increases ghrelin which is a hormone that increases appetite. Studies have also shown that chronic sleep deprivation is associated with an increased risk of obesity and diabetes. In the 15 year long Massachusetts Male Aging Study (MMAS) showed that male subjects who self-reported less than 6 hours of sleep were twice as likely to develop diabetes. [66]

The American College of Sports Medicine (ACSM) reports that adults who get less than seven to eight hours of sleep may feel sluggish or lack energy and motivation to exercise. However, ACSM also reports that partaking in a morning workout (7 a.m.) "invoked significantly greater improvements in quality of sleep versus exercising later in the day (1 p.m. and 7 p.m.).[67] But those with high blood pressure may want to avoid early morning workouts, as blood pressure tends to rise slightly for all of us after waking. For those with high blood pressure, this elevation may persist longer with early morning exercise.

As you can see, it is still highly recommended that 7-8 hours of sleep be attained for adults.

Conclusion: Myth

APPENDIX

Instructions for use of the Macronutrient/Calories Worksheet.

This worksheet can be used for each meal consumed during each day. You can use this worksheet to help you to gauge the amount of fats, protein and carbohydrates that you typically eat for each meal.

- Add each food item that you plan to eat for each meal. For example, breakfast may include, eggs, oatmeal, bread and orange juice.
- Determine the number of grams per serving for each macronutrient. As shown in the example on the next page, a typical chicken breast contains 30 grams of carbohydrates, 6 grams of fat, 20 grams of protein and 7 grams of fiber.
- Determine how many servings you will have for each item.
- Multiply the number of servings by the grams for each macronutrient. For example, corn has 20 grams of carbohydrates per serving. Since 2 servings of corn will be consumed, the total number of grams of carbohydrates is 40 grams of carbohydrates for 2 servings and so on. (4 grams of fat x 2 servings = 8 grams).
- Add the totals for macronutrient.
- Calculate the total number of calories for each macronutrient. (reminder-4 calories for each gram of carbohydrate and protein and 9 calories for each gram of fat) Subtract from the total calories for carbohydrates, any calories for fiber over 5 grams
- Determine the % makeup for each macronutrient. (For example 262 calories (carbohydrates)/ 474 total calories=55%.
- Compare your total daily macronutrient % breakdown to ACSM's macronutrient recommendations.
- Make as many copies of the sample worksheets, as needed.

** Compare the TDEE that you calculated for yourself to the total daily calories. Are you above or below your calculated TDEE?

Sample Macronutrient/Calories Worksheet

Instruction steps	Meal/Snack	Name of Food	Carbohydrates grams/serving	Fat (grams/serving)	Protein (grams/serving)	Fiber* (grams/serving)	# of servings
	Item 1	Chicken Breast	30	6	20	7	1
	Item 2	Corn	40	8	4	0	2
	Item 3						
1, 2, 3, 4	Item 4						
	Item 5						
	Item 6						
	Beverage					Total	
5	Total daily grams		70	14	24	7	
6	Total daily calories**		280-28(fiber)=262	126	96	(28)	474
7	Total daily macronutrient %		55%	27%	20%		
8	ACSM recommendation		45%-65%	20%-35%	10%-35%		

*Fiber-5 grams or more of fiber can be subtracted from the total grams or calories of carbohydrates.
**Compare to TDEE calculation.

Sample Macronutrient/Calories Worksheet

Instruction steps	Meal/Snack	Name of Food	Carbohydrates grams/serving	Fat (grams/serving)	Protein (grams/serving)	Fiber* (grams/serving)	# of servings
1, 2, 3, 4							
	Total						
5	Total daily grams						
6	Total daily calories**						
7	Total daily macronutrient %						
8	ACSM recommendation		45%-65%	20%-35%	10%-35%		

*Fiber-5 grams or more of fiber can be subtracted from the total grams or calories of carbohydrates.
**Compare to TDEE calculation.

Sample Health History Questionnaire

You have had:

___ a definite or suspected heart attack or stroke

___ heart surgery or coronary bypass surgery

___ cardiac catheterization

___ coronary angioplasty (PTCA)

___ pacemaker/implantable cardiac

___ defibrillator/rhythm disturbance

___ heart valve disease

___ heart failure

___ heart transplantation

___ congenital heart disease

___ cardiovascular or pulmonary (lung) disease

___ You experience chest discomfort with exertion.

___ You experience shortness of breath

___ You have a known heart murmur.

___ You have pain in the legs that causes you to stop walking (claudication)

___ You experience unreasonable breathlessness.

___ You experience dizziness, fainting, or blackouts.

___ You take heart medications.

If you marked any of these statements in this section, consult your physician or other appropriate health care provider before engaging in exercise. You may need to use an exercise facility with a medically qualified staff.

Other health issues

___ You have diabetes.

___ You have thyroid, kidney or liver disease

___ You have asthma or other lung disease.

___ You have burning or cramping sensation in your lower legs when walking short distances.

___ You have musculoskeletal problems that limit your physical activity.

___ You have concerns about the safety of exercise.

___ You take prescription medication(s).

___ You are pregnant.

___ You take high blood pressure medications or within the last 12 months have taken medication to control your blood pressure

If you marked any of these statements in this section, consult your physician or other appropriate health care provider before engaging in exercise. You may need to use a facility with a medically qualified staff.

Cardiovascular risk factors

___ You are a man older than 45 years.

___ You are a woman older than 55 years, have had a hysterectomy, or are postmenopausal.

___ You smoke, or quit smoking within the previous 6 months.

___ Your blood pressure is >140/90 mm Hg.

___ You do not know your blood pressure.

___ You take blood pressure medication.

___ Your blood cholesterol level is > 200 mg/dL.

___ You do not know your cholesterol level.

___ You have a close blood relative who had a heart attack or heart surgery before age 55 (father or brother) or age 65 (mother or sister).

___ You are physically inactive (i.e., you get <30 minutes of physical activity on at least 3 days per week).

___ You are > 20 pounds overweight.

___ You have an impaired fasting blood glucose greater than or equal to 100 mg/dL but less than 126 mg/dL or an impaired glucose tolerance test greater than or equal to 140 mg/dL but less than 200 mg/Dl.

___ You have a low density lipoprotein of greater than or equal to 130 mg/dL or a high density lipoprotein of less than 40 mg/dL or on lipid lowering medication.

If you marked two or more of the statements in this section, you should consult your physician or other appropriate health care provider before engaging in exercise. You might benefit from using a facility with a professionally qualified exercise staff to guide your exercise program.

Sample
BEHAVIOR CONTRACT

A position statement given by the American College of Sports Medicine recommends that all adults need to exercise 3-5 times per week for 20-90 minutes of continuous or intermittent aerobic exercise at 64-94% their maximum heart rate in order to develop and maintain adult fitness. Activities which provide rhythmic movement of the large muscle groups include swimming, biking, running, jogging, walking, aerobic exercise classes, rowing, and some select sports.

I_____, agree to adhere to at least an   week exercise program which complies with the American College of Sports Medicine's recommendations.

___I agree to follow the aerobic and/or anaerobic program created by

_____

___I agree that I will celebrate each success no matter how small.

___I agree that I understand that this is a long term process and I will commit myself fully to this process of improving my overall physical
     well-being.

____ I understand that I can refer to the Seven Rules for Fitness Success and Behavior Change Model for help to reach my fitness goals.

___I agree that I will report my activities accordingly to my contract witness(es) for his/her/their signatures weekly.

Participant's signature_____

I,_____, agree to act as a contract witness and encourage and sign off on the weekly exercise progress of the above participant only in the case of ideal adherence.
Contract Witness
Signature_____

I,_____, agree to act as a contract witness and encourage and sign off on the weekly exercise progress of the above participant only in the case of ideal adherence.
Contract Witness
Signature_____

I,_____, agree to act as a contract witness and encourage and sign off on the weekly exercise progress of the above participant only in the case of ideal adherence.
Contract Witness
Signature_____

Sample Resistance Training Program
Week 1-2

Day 1	Sets	Intensity	Reps	Day 2	Sets	Intensity	Reps	Day 3	Sets	Intensity	Reps
Warm-up				Warm-up				Warm-up			
Bench press	3		10-12	Bench press	3		10-12	Bench press	3		10-12
Lateral Pulldown	3		10-12	Lateral Pulldown	3		10-12	Lateral Pulldown	3		10-12
Leg Press	3		10-12	Leg Press	3		10-12	Leg Press	3		10-12
Shoulder press	3		10-12	Shoulder press	3		10-12	Shoulder press	3		10-12
EZ Curl Barl	3		10-12	Dumbbell curl	3		10-12	Dumbbell curl	3		10-12
Tricep extension	3		10-12	Tricep extension	3		10-12	Tricep extension	3		10-12
Seated calf raise	3		12-15	Seated calf raise	3		12-15	Seated calf raise	3		12-15
Crunch	3		15-20	Crunch	3		15-20	Crunch	3		15-20
Cool-down	5 mins			Cool-down	5 mins			Cool-down	5 mins		
Stretch				Stretch				Stretch			

Rest period between sets should be no more than 2-3 minutes.
You can take develop a circuit training program with the exercises listed above by reducing the rest period between each set to 20 seconds or 30 seconds.

Basic Total Body Resistance Program for Beginners

Sample Resistance Training Program
Week 3-4

Day 1	Sets	Intensity	Reps	Day 2	Sets	Intensity	Reps	Day 3	Sets	Intensity	Reps
Warm-up				Warm-up				Warm-up			
Bench press	3		10-12	Bench press	3		10-12	Bench press	3		10-12
Lateral Pulldown	3		10-12	Lateral Pulldown	3		10-12	Lateral Pulldown	3		10-12
Leg Press	3		10-12	Leg Press	3		10-12	Leg Press	3		10-12
Shoulder press	3		10-12	Shoulder press	3		10-12	Shoulder press	3		10-12
EZ Curl Bar	3		10-12	Dumbbell curl	3		10-12	Dumbbell curl	3		10-12
Tricep extension	3		10-12	Tricep extension	3		10-12	Tricep extension	3		10-12
Seated calf raise	3		12-15	Seated calf raise	3		12-15	Seated calf raise	3		12-15
Crunch	3		15-20	Crunch	3		15-20	Crunch	3		15-20
Cool-down				Cool-down				Cool-down			
Stretch				Stretch				Stretch			

177

Sample Resistance Training Program
Week 1-2

Day 1	Sets	Intensity	Reps	Day 2	Sets	Intensity	Reps	Day 3	Sets	Intensity	Reps
Warm-up				Warm-up				Warm-up			
Flat Bench press	3		10-12	Squat	3		10-12	Lateral Pulldown	3		10-12
Incline press	3		10-12	Leg press	3		10-12	One-arm dumbbell row	3 x 2		10-12
Decline press	3		10-12	Seated leg extension	3		10-12	Low-row pulley machine	3		10-12
Tricep extension	3		10-12	Seated leg curl	3		10-12	EZ Curl Bar (standing)	3		10-12
Tricep dip machine	3		10-12	Barbell lunge	3		10-12	Alternating dumbbell Hammer curl (standing)	3 x 2		10-12
Close grip bench	3		10-12	Seated Hip abduction	3		10-12	Incline Alternating Dumbbell Curl	3 x 2		10-12
Cable kickback	3 x 2		12-15	Seated Calf raise machine	3		12-15	Crunch	3		12-15
Crunch	3		20-25	Russian twist	3		15-20	Scissor Kick	3		15-20
Cool-down				Cool-down				Cool-down			
Stretch				Stretch				Stretch			

Rest period between sets should be no more than 2-3 minutes.

Basic Circuit Training program-You can take develop a circuit training program with the exercises listed above by reducing the rest period between each set to 20 seconds or 30 seconds.

Basic muscle building program-To make this program into a muscle building program, reduce the repetitions to 6-10 and increase the intensity each week by 5% to 10%. For example, the intensity for week 1-2 should be raised from 60% to 65% or 70% and week 3-4 should be raised from 70% to 75% or 80%. Weeks 5-6 should include at least 1 set of intensities of 100% to 110% of 1RM for each muscle group worked.(Be sure to use a spotter.)

Sample Resistance Training Program
Week 3-4

Day 1	Sets	Intensity	Reps	Day 2	Sets	Intensity	Reps	Day 3	Sets	Intensity	Reps
Warm-up											
Flat Bench press	3	70%or 70lbs	10-12	Squat	3	70% or 105lbs	10-12	Lateral Pulldown	3	70% or 56lbs	10-12
Incline press	3	70%x 67lbs	10-12	Leg press	3	70% or 140lbs	10-12	One-arm dumbbell row	3 x 2	70% or 25lbs	10-12
Decline press	3	70%or 77lbs	10-12	Seated leg extension	3	70% or 42lbs	10-12	Low-row pulley machine	3	70% or 56lbs	10-12
Tricep extension	3	70%or 25lbs	10-12	Seated leg curl	3	70% or 42lbs	10-12	EZ Curl Bar (standing)	3	70% or 25lbs	10-12
Tricep dip machine	3	70%x 24lbs	10-12	Barbell lunge	3	70% or 49lbs	10-12	Alternating dumbbell Hammer curl (standing)	3 x 2	70% or 14lbs	10-12
Close grip bench	3	70%x 63lb	10-12	Seated Hip abduction	3	70% or 84lbs	10-12	Incline Alternating Dumbbell Curl	3 x 2	70% or 14lbs	10-12
Cable kickback	3 x 2	70% 25lbs	12-15	Seated Calf raise machine	3	70% or 70lbs	12-15	Crunch	3	20-25	12-15
Crunch	3		20-25	Russian twist	3	10lbs ball/dumbbell	15-20	Scissor Kick	3	30 secs	15-20
Cool-down		5 mins		Cool-down		5 mins		Cool-down		5 mins	
Stretch				Stretch				Stretch			

Sample Resistance Band Training Program
Week 1-2

Day 1	Sets	Intensity	Reps
Warm-up Jog in place/jumping jacks	1	5-6 minutes	
Push-up	3		10-12
Standing Chest press	3		10-12
Narrow-width push-up	3		10-12
Tricep kickback	3		10-12
Overhead tricep extension	3		10-12
Kneeling crunch	3		10-12
Woodchoppers	3 x 2		12-15
Reverse crunch	3		20-25
Cool-down	5 mins		
Stretch			

Day 2	Sets	Intensity	Reps
Warm-up Jog in place/jumping jacks	1	5-6 minutes	
Front Squat	3		10-12
Leg extension	3		10-12
Prone leg curl	3		10-12
Standing or seated abduction	3		10-12
Lunge	3		10-12
Toe raises	3		10-12
Russian twist	3		12-15
Kneeling crunch	3		15-20
Cool-down	5 mins		
Stretch			

Day 3	Sets	Intensity	Reps
Warm-up Jog in place/jumping jacks	1	5-6 minutes	
Lateral pulldown	3		10-12
Bent over row	3 x 2		10-12
Overhead press	3		10-12
Lateral raise	3		10-12
Upright row	3 x 2		10-12
Standing bicep curl	3 x 2		10-12
Concentration curl	3		12-15
Russian twist	3		15-20
Cool-down	5 mins		
Stretch			

Workout for at Home or Outdoor Use Using Resistance Bands

Sample Resistance Band Training Program
Week 3-4

Day 1	Sets	Intensity	Reps	Day 2	Sets	Intensity	Reps	Day 3	Sets	Intensity	Reps
Warm-up Jog in place/jumping jacks	1	5-6 minutes		Warm-up Jog in place/jumping jacks	1	5-6 minutes					
Push-up	3		10-12	Front Squat	3		10-12	Lateral pulldown	3		10-12
Standing Chest press	3		10-12	Leg extension	3		10-12	Bent over row	3 x 2		10-12
Narrow-width push-up	3		10-12	Prone leg curl	3		10-12	Overhead press	3		10-12
Tricep kickback	3		10-12	Standing or seated abduction	3		10-12	Lateral raise	3		10-12
Overhead tricep extension	3		10-12	Lunge	3		10-12	Upright row	3 x 2		10-12
Kneeling crunch	3		10-12	Toe raises	3		10-12	Standing bicep curl	3 x 2		10-12
Woodchoppers	3 x 2		12-15	Russian twist	3		12-15	Concentration curl	3		12-15
Reverse crunch	3		20-25	Kneeling crunch	3		15-20	Russian twist	3		15-20
Cool-down	5 mins			Cool-down	5 mins			Cool-down	5 mins		
Stretch				Stretch				Stretch			

Resources

Basal Energy calculator
http://www.mdcalc.com/basal-energy-expenditure/

Checking your resting heart rate-Video
https://www.youtube.com/watch?v=vpLXTpiVUys

CVS Minute Clinic
www.cvs.com/minuteclinic

Glycemic Index
http://www.glycemicindex.com/

Katch-McArdle Calculator
http://www.burnthefatinnercircle.com/members/Katch-McArdle-Calorie-Calculator-For-Men-And-Women.cfm

Lab Test online
http://labtestsonline.org/

Mental Health
http://www.mentalhealth.gov/

http://www.mentalhealthamerica.net/finding-therapy

Organic foods vs Conventional foods
http://www.webmd.com/food-recipes/organic-food-better

Satiety
http://nutritiondata.self.com/topics/fullness-factor

SilverSneakers
https://www.silversneakers.com/

Walgreen's Clinic
http://www.walgreens.com/topic/pharmacy/healthcare-clinic.jsp

Walmart Clinic
http://www.walmart.com/cp/Walmart-Clinics
United States Registry of Exercise Professionals
https://usrepsmember.goamp.com/Net/USREPSWcm/Membership/Directory/Shar
ed_Content/Directory.aspx

USDA Food Plans: Cost of Food Plans
http://www.cnpp.usda.gov/USDAFoodPlansCostofFood/reports

Yoga
http://www.yogafinder.com/

References

1. Fryar, Cheryl D., Margaret D. Carroll, and Cynthia L. Ogden. "Obesity and Overweight." *Centers for Disease Control and Prevention*. Centers for Disease Control and Prevention, 30 Sept. 2015. Web. 12 Oct. 2015.
2. "Cardiovascular Diseases (CVDs)." *WHO*. N.p., Jan. 2015. Web. 12 Oct. 2015.
3. Alagiakrishnan, Kannayiram, and Anita Chopra. "*Health and Health Care of Asian Indian American.*" Health and Health Care of Asian Indian American. N.p., n.d. Web. 12 Oct. 2015.
4. "Recommendations for Preventing Osteoporosis." *World Health Organization* (n.d.): n. pag. Web.12Oct.2015.<http://www.who.int/dietphysicalactivity/publications/trs916/en/gsfao _osteo.pdf>.
5. Cauley, JA. "Result Filters." *National Center for Biotechnology Information*. U.S. National Library of Medicine, n.d. Web. 12 Oct. 2015.
6. "Heart Disease Facts." *Centers for Disease Control and Prevention*. Centers for Disease Control and Prevention, 10 Aug. 2015. Web. 12 Oct. 2015. <http://www.cdc.gov/heartdisease/facts.htm>.
7. "Statistics About Diabetes." *American Diabetes Association*. N.p., n.d. Web. 12 Oct. 2015. <http://www.diabetes.org/diabetes-basics/statistics/?referrer=https%3A%2F%2Fwww.google.com%2F>.
8. "Osteoporosis." *Risk Factors*. N.p., n.d. Web. 12 Oct. 2015. <http://www.mayoclinic.org/diseases-conditions/osteoporosis/basics/risk-factors/con-20019924>.
9. "Life Expectancy." *Centers for Disease Control and Prevention*. Centers for Disease Control and Prevention, 29 Apr. 2015. Web. 12 Oct. 2015. <http://www.cdc.gov/nchs/fastats/life-expectancy.htm>.
10. "The State of Obesity." *Special Report: Racial and Ethnic Disparities in Obesity*. N.p., n.d. Web. 12 Oct. 2015. <http://www.stateofobesity.org/disparities>.
11. Brennan Ramirez LK, Baker EA, Metzler M. Promoting Health Equity: A Resource to Help Communities Address Social Determinants of Health. Atlanta: U.S. Department of Health and Human Services, Centers for Disease Control and Prevention; 2008.
12. Holt, Susanna, JC Miller, P. Petocz, and E. Farmakalidis. "Result Filters." *National Center for Biotechnology Information*. U.S. National Library of Medicine, n.d. Web. 12 Oct. 2015. <http://www.ncbi.nlm.nih.gov/pubmed/7498104>.

13. Albers, Susan. *50 Ways to Soothe Yourself without Food*. Oakland, CA: New Harbinger Publications, 2009. Print.

14. Wing, RR, and RW Jefferey. "Benefits of Recruiting Participants with Friends and Increasing Social Support for Weight Loss and Maintenance." *National Center for Biotechnology Information*. U.S. National Library of Medicine, Feb. 1999. Web. 12 Oct. 2015. <http://www.ncbi.nlm.nih.gov/pubmed/10028217>.

15. Williams, Ray. "Good Looks Will Get You That Job, Promotion and Raise." *Psychology Today*. N.p., n.d. Web. 12 Oct. 2015. <https://www.psychologytoday.com/blog/wired-success/201109/good-looks-will-get-you-job-promotion-and-raise>.

16. "Sleep Deprivation Fosters Inactivity." *ACSM | ACSM in the News*. N.p., n.d. Web. 12 Oct. 2015.

17. Makino, Maria, Koji Tsuboi, and Lorraine Dennerstein. "Prevalence of Eating Disorders: A Comparison of Western and Non-Western Countries." *Medscape General Medicine*. Medscape, n.d. Web. 12 Oct. 2015.

18. "For Best Sleep, Work Up a Sweat in the Morning." *ACSM | ACSM in the News*. N.p., 01 Aug. 2011. Web. 17 Oct. 2015. <http://www.acsm.org/about-acsm/media-room/acsm-in-the-news/2011/08/01/for-best-sleep-work-up-a-sweat-in-the-morning>.

19. Makino, Maria, Koji Tsuboi, and Lorraine Dennerstein. "Prevalence of Eating Disorders: A Comparison of Western and Non-Western Countries." *Medscape General Medicine*. Medscape, 27 Sept. 2004. Web. 17 Oct. 2015. <http://www.ncbi.nlm.nih.gov/pmc/articles/PMC1435625/>.

20. Bowen, R. "*Gastrointestinal Transit*." Gastrointestinal Transit. N.p., 27 May 2006. Web. 17 Oct. 2015. <http://www.vivo.colostate.edu/hbooks/pathphys/digestion/basics/transit.html>.

21. McMillan, Beverly. "Digestive System: Oral Disorders." *The Illustrated Atlas of the Human Body*. Hamburg: Argosy, 2011. 182. Print. Copyright Weldon Owen Pty Ltd

22. McMillan, Beverly. "Digestive System: Oral Disorders." *The Illustrated Atlas of the Human Body*. Hamburg: Argosy, 2011. 185. Print. Copyright Weldon Owen Pty Ltd

23. McMillan, Beverly. "Digestive System: Oral Disorders." *The Illustrated Atlas of the Human Body*. Hamburg: Argosy, 2011. 178. Print. Copyright Weldon Owen Pty Ltd

24. McMillan, Beverly. "Digestive System: The Small and Large Intestines." *The Illustrated Atlas of the Human Body*. Hamburg: Argosy, 2011. 178-179. Print. Copyright Weldon Owen Pty Ltd

25. Ballentine, Jerry. "Pancreatitis: Click for Symptoms, Diet, and Treatments." *MedicineNet*. N.p., n.d. Web. 18 Oct. 2015. <http://www.medicinenet.com/pancreatitis/article.htm>.

26. "Type 2." *American Diabetes Association*. N.p., n.d. Web. 18 Oct. 2015. <http://www.diabetes.org/diabetes-basics/type-2/?referrer=https%3A%2F%2Fwww.google.com%2F>.

27. Rae-Dupree, Janet, and Pat DuPree. *Anatomy & Physiology Workbook for Dummies*. Hoboken, NJ: Wiley Pub., 2007. Print.

28. Delavier, Frédéric. *Women's Strength Training Anatomy*. Champaign, IL: Human Kinetics, 2003. Print.

29. Hyman, MD Mark. "Are You a Skinny Fat Person? 10 Steps to Cure the Skinny Fat Syndrome." *The Huffington Post*. TheHuffingtonPost.com, n.d. Web. 18 Oct. 2015. <http://www.huffingtonpost.com/dr-mark-hyman/skinny-fat_b_1799797.html>.

30. "ACSM Body Fat Guidelines." *LIVESTRONG.COM*. LIVESTRONG.COM, 06 June 2015. Web. 18 Oct. 2015. <http://www.livestrong.com/article/426250-acsm-body-fat-guidelines/>.

31. Berggren, Jason, Matthew Hulver, and Joseph Houmard. "Fat as an Endocrine Organ: Influence of Exercise." *Journal of Applied Physiology*. N.p., 1 Aug. 2005. Web. 18 Oct. 2015. <http://jap.physiology.org/content/99/2/757>.

32. Powers, Scott K., and Edward T. Howley. *Exercise Physiology: Theory and Application to Fitness and Performance*. Boston: McGraw-Hill, 2007. Print.

33. Mozzaffarian, Dariush, Tao Hoa, Eric Rimm, Walter C. Willett, and Frank Hu. "Changes in Diet and Lifestyle and Long-Term Weight Gain in Women and Men — NEJM." *New England Journal of Medicine*. N.p., 23 June 2011. Web. 18 Oct. 2015. <http://www.nejm.org/doi/full/10.1056/NEJMoa1014296>.

34. "Glycemic Index." *University of Sydney Glycemic Index*. N.p., n.d. Web. 18 Oct. 2015. <http://www.glycemicindex.com/>.

35. Sapolsky, Robert. "How the Brain Uses Glucose to Fuel Self-Control." *Wall Street Journal*. N.p., 3 Dec. 2014. Web. 18 Oct. 2015. <http://www.wsj.com/articles/how-the-brain-uses-glucose-to-fuel-self-control-1417618996>.

36. Wong, Stephen. "GLYCEMIC INDEX AND GLYCEMIC LOAD: Their Application in Healt... : ACSM's Health & Fitness Journal." *American College of Sports Medicine*. N.p., Nov.-Dec. 2010.Web.18Oct.2015.<http://journals.lww.com/acsm-healthfitness/Fulltext/2010/11000/GLYCEMIC_INDEX_AND_GLYCEMIC_LOAD__Their.7.aspx>.

37. Stoppani, Jim. "Wet Your Whistle While You Workout." *Muscle and Performance* Oct. 2012: 55-57. Web. 18 Oct. 2015.

38. Karp, Jason, Jeanne Johnston, Sandra Tecklenburg, Timothy Mickleborough, and Joel Stanger. "Got Chocolate Milk for Exercise Recovery?" *The Physician and Sportsmedicine Phy Sportsmed* 32.7 (2004): 0. *International Journal of Sport Nutrition and Exercise Metabolism*. 2006. Web. 18 Oct. 2015.

39. Stoppani, Jim. "Everything You Need to Know About Protein." Men's Fitness. N.p., n.d. Web. 18 Oct. 2015. <http://www.mensfitness.com/nutrition/supplements/everything-you-need-to-know-about-protein>.

40. Cataldo, Donna. "Protein Intake for Optimal Muscle Maintenance." *ACSM Information On... PROTEIN INTAKE FOR OPTIMAL MUSCLE MAINTENANCE* (n.d.): n. pag. 2015. Web. 18 Oct. 2015.

41. Berg, Michael, and Carey Rossi. "Protein Powder." *Muscle and Performance* Sept. 2009: 36-40. Web. 18 Oct. 2015.

42. "What Is a Protein's Biological Value and Why Is It Important?" *Foodeducate*. N.p., 12 Nov. 2014. Web. 18 Oct. 2015. <http://blog.fooducate.com/2014/11/12/what-is-a-proteins-biological-value-and-why-is-it-important/>.

43. "Monounsaturated Fats." *American Heart Association: Monounsaturated Fats*. N.p., 7 Oct. 2015. Web. 18 Oct. 2015. <http://www.heart.org/HEARTORG/GettingHealthy/NutritionCenter/HealthyEating/Mo nounsaturated-Fats_UCM_301460_Article.jsp#.ViQbRfmrTcs>.

44. "Polyunsaturated Fats." *American Heart Association: Polyunsaturated Fats*. N.p., 7 Oct. 2015. Web. 18 Oct. 2015. <http://www.heart.org/HEARTORG/GettingHealthy/NutritionCenter/HealthyEating/Pol yunsaturated-Fats_UCM_301461_Article.jsp#.ViQaz_mrTcs>.

45. "Nutrition and Healthy Eating." *Trans Fat: A Double Whammy*. N.p., 26 Feb. 2013. Web. 18 Oct. 2015. <http://www.mayoclinic.org/healthy-lifestyle/nutrition-and-healthy-eating/in-depth/health-tip/art-20049258>.

46. "Daily Values." *National Institutes of Health (DVs)*. N.p., n.d. Web. 18 Oct. 2015. <https://ods.od.nih.gov/HealthInformation/dailyvalues.aspx>.

47. "Portion Size Plate | Recommended Serving Sizes for Portion Control." *WebMD*. WebMD, n.d. Web. 18 Oct. 2015.

48. "Super Size Me." *Wikipedia*. Wikimedia Foundation, n.d. Web. 18 Oct. 2015.

49. Drake, Meghan. "Appeals Court Closes Door on Bloomberg's 'Soda Ban'; Tony Gwynn's Cancer Death Could Help E-Cigarettes Substitute for Tobacco." *The Washington Times (Washington, DC)*. N.p., 27 June 2014. Web. 18 Oct. 2015.

50. "*USDA Food Plans: Cost of Food*: March 2015." USDA Food Plans: Cost of Food. N.p., Mar. 2015. Web. 18 Oct. 2015.

51. "*Visa Survey Shows Americans Doling Out $936 Annually for Lunch Out.*" Visa Survey Shows Americans Doling Out $936 Annually for Lunch Out. N.p., n.d. Web. 18 Oct. 2015.

52. "*Statistic Brain*: Gym Membership Statistics." Statistic Brain. N.p., n.d. Web. 18 Oct. 2015.

53. Zipes, Douglas P., and Hein Wellens. "Sudden Cardiac Death." *American Heart Association: Clinical Cardiology: New Frontiers* (n.d.): n. pag. Web. <http://circ.ahajournals.org/content/98/21/2334.full>.

54. "Death by Exercise." *Men's Health*. Ed. Lou Schuler. N.p., 8 June 2003. Web. 18 Oct. 2015.

55. Zink, AJ, WC Whiting, and AJ Mclaine. "The Effects of a Weight Belt on Trunk and Leg Muscle Activity and Joint Kinematics during the Squat Exercise." *National Center for Biotechnology Information*. U.S. National Library of Medicine, 15 May 2001. Web. 18 Oct. 2015.

56. Bushman, Barbara Ann. *Complete Guide to Fitness & Health*. Champaign, IL: Human Kinetics, 2011. Print.

57. Stoppani, James. *Encyclopedia of Muscle & Strength*. Champaign, IL: Human Kinetics, 2006. Print.

58. Levine, JA. "Non Exercise Activity Thermogenesis." *National Center for Biotechnology Information*. U.S. National Library of Medicine, 16 Dec. 2002. Web. 18 Oct. 2015.

59. "The FITTE Factor." *SUNY Downstate Medical Center: Controling Obesity*. N.p., n.d. Web. 18 Oct. 2015.

60. "Patellofemoral Pain Syndrome-Topic Overview." *WebMD*. WebMD, n.d. Web. 18 Oct. 2015.

61. "Testosterone Levels by Age." *Healthline*. N.p., n.d. Web. 18 Oct. 2015.

62. "Ketoacidosis." *MedicineNet*. N.p., n.d. Web. 18 Oct. 2015.

63. Thiebaud, Robert. *Exercise Induced Muscle Damage; Is It Detrimental or Beneficial?* San Diego, CA: Greenhaven, 1996. Journal of Trainology. Web. 18 Oct. 2015.

64. "Delayed Onset Muscle Soreness." *American College of Sports Medicine* (2011): n. pag. *American College of Sports Medicine*. 2011. Web. 18 Oct. 2015.

65. Schoenfeld, BJ. "Result Filters." *National Center for Biotechnology Information*. U.S. National Library of Medicine, 1 Dec. 2012. Web. 19 Oct. 2015. <http://www.ncbi.nlm.nih.gov/pubmed/23013520>.

66. Sharma, Sunil, and Mani Kavuru. "Sleep and Metabolism: An Overview." *International Journal of Endocrinology*. Hindawi Publishing Corporation, 2 Aug. 2010. Web. 19 Oct. 2015. <http://www.ncbi.nlm.nih.gov/pmc/articles/PMC2929498/>.

67. "For Best Sleep, Work Up a Sweat in the Morning." *ACSM | ACSM in the News*.

68. Smith, A. (2000). Introduction-Robert Reich. In The wealth of nations (pp. 17-18). New
    York: Random House International.

69. National Healthcare Quality & Disparities Reports. (2014). Retrieved December 7, 2015,
    from http://www.ahrq.gov/research/findings/nhqrdr/index.html

70. Thomas, D., & Frankenberg, E. (2002). Health, Nutrition and Prosperity: A microeconomic
    perspective. Retrieved December 7, 2015, from
    http://www.who.int/bulletin/archives/80(2)106.pdf

The Owner's Manual for Health and Fitness

This step-by-step manual was developed to help people from all walks of life to achieve their health and fitness goals.

Over 58 million, very diverse people, across the country hold gym memberships. Worldwide, even more diverse people, who do not have access to a fitness facility, seek to reach their health and fitness aims. Unfortunately, an information gap exists that limits people from reaching their goals. Most are not equipped with the necessary health and fitness information to guide them and others don't have access to health and fitness professionals who can help them. Professional athlete, American College of Sports Medicine Certified Trainer and National Academy of Sports Medicine Weight Loss Specialist, George Dorsey, created this manual to fill this information gap and to provide to everyone, the techniques, strategies and tools that health and fitness professionals use to create the most effective physical fitness programs. This manual includes:

- The Seven Rules for Fitness Success;

- Behavior Change Model;

- Tools and information to help reduce the risk for diabetes, high blood pressure, cardiovascular disease and other preventable diseases;

- Tools and tips on the proper methods to lose weight and to build muscle mass;

- Information on the various types of protein, carbohydrates and fats;

- Tools to help you decide which type of fitness equipment you need the most;

- Information to help you to accurately read a food label; determine if specific food is right for you;

- Step-by-step details to help you to develop your own cardiorespiratory (aerobic) exercise program;

- Step-by-step details to help you to develop your own resistance training (anaerobic) exercise program;

- Information to dispel the most common health and fitness myths.

About the Author

For over 20 years, IFBB Pro George Dorsey, ACSM-CPT, NASM-Weight Loss Specialist (WLS), has been helping people to reach their health and fitness goals. As an Advisory Board member, George provides guidance to a multi-million-dollar health and fitness company. George also writes for a health and fitness blog and is sometimes quoted in national print media. George has two loves; Diversity and Fitness. As a Diversity Consultant, George worked with Fortune 500 companies, and local and state government to develop large scale diversity initiatives. He has also worked with a New York Times Best Selling Author to enhance MGM/Mirage's Diversity Initiative. In this book, George is able to merge his two loves by providing relevant health and fitness information to people from all walks of life. George has lived in 6 different states encompassing the east and west coast. He has roots in Charlotte, N.C. and Baltimore, M.D. He currently resides in Gwinnett County, GA. He serves part-time as a military officer in the Air Force Reserves. Even after turning 40, he continues to epitomize the notion that we keep getting better with age.

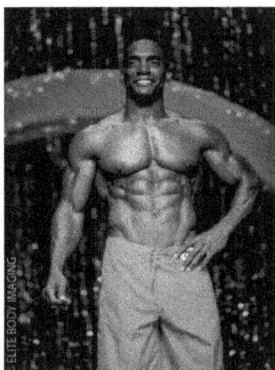

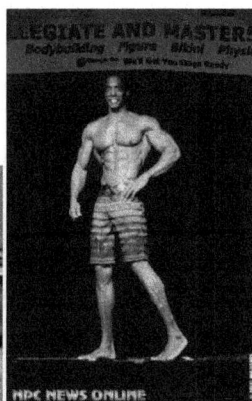

George's Mom
Marilyn Dorsey

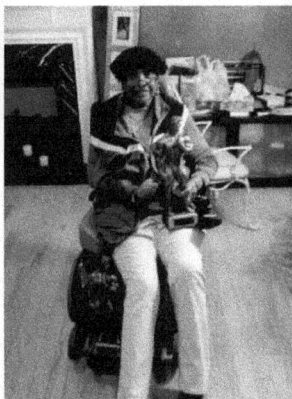

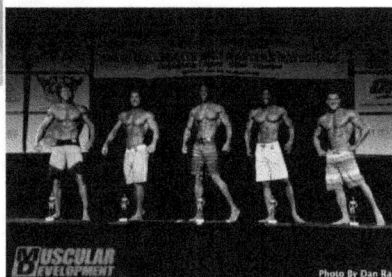

Winning his IFBB Pro Card

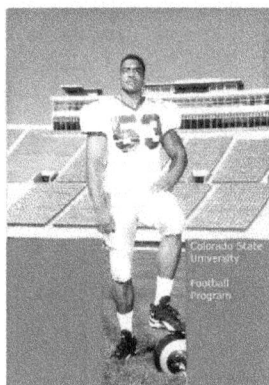

Defensive End
Colorado State University

www.ingramcontent.com/pod-product-compliance
Lightning Source LLC
Chambersburg PA
CBHW081151270326
41930CB00014B/3113